LIVING WITH HEAD INJURY
A GUIDE FOR FAMILIES

by
Richard C. Senelick, M.D.
and
Cathy E. Ryan

This book is not intended to replace personal medical care and/or professional supervision; there is no substitute for the experience and information that your doctor or health professional can provide. Rather, it is our hope that this book will provide additional information to help people understand the nature of head injury and its effects on its victims and their families.

Proper treatment should always be tailored to the individual. If you read something in this book that seems to conflict with your doctor or health professional's instructions, contact him/her. There may be sound reasons for recommending treatment that may differ from the information presented in this book.

If you have any questions about any treatment in this book, please consult your doctor or health care professional.

In addition, the names and cases used in this book do not represent actual people, but are composite cases drawn from several sources.

Facts About Rehab Hospital of York

Opened in 1983, the Rehab Hospital of York offers comprehensive physical rehabilitation. With 88 beds and a staff of over 300 rehabilitation specialists, the hospital provides patients with a strong professional staff-to-patient ratio. We use a wellness approach in a normalized environment. The new, modern facilities offer patients a bright, warm environment for healing and recovery, yet one where the rehabilitation process is intensely pursued.

We develop individualized programs on both an inpatient and outpatient basis. We pride ourselves on our ability to develop close working relationships with everyone concerned—the patient, the family, physicians and others.

The Rehab Hospital is located in York, Pennsylvania, approximately 50 miles north of Baltimore and 25 miles south of Harrisburg. We serve the needs of patients in Pennsylvania, Maryland, West Virginia, Washington, D.C. and surrounding states.

The Head Injury Program at Rehab Hospital of York is recognized by the independent nonprofit Commission on Accreditation of Rehabilitation Facilities (CARF) as complying with national standards in all aspects of quality care. Rehab Hospital of York has earned three-year accreditation in:

—Acute Head Injury (Inpatient Program)
—Post-acute Head Injury (Day Rehab Program)
—Comprehensive Inpatient Rehab
—Spinal Cord Injury
—Chronic Pain Management (Incentives)
—Work Hardening Programs (The Work Station)

We're ready to help you achieve the best possible future. Call today for information or assistance at 717-767-6941.

Acknowledgments

A special thanks goes to Karla Dougherty of PIA Press whose help, assistance and guidance was invaluable. Karla's unbounding enthusiasm and literary skills were instrumental in bringing this book to life. Finally, we would like to thank Mr. Bradly Anderson, Chief Executive Officer of the Rehabilitation Institute of San Antonio. His unflagging support of clinical excellence and education has provided an environment in which projects such as this book may flourish.

Dedication

This book is dedicated to the patients and families who have had to endure the tragedy of head injury. It is through them that we have learned so much both intellectually and emotionally. They endure on a minute to minute and hour to hour basis those things that we all hope we will never have to face. We have never walked in their shoes nor had to sit in their chairs, but we hope that our collective experience in dealing with Head Injury Rehabilitation will help families adjust to a new way of life and deal with the difficult issues and challenges that arise on a daily basis. We are constantly amazed at the strength and adaptability of the human spirit and the day to day strength that is shown to us by the families of our head injured survivors.

CONTENTS

INTRODUCTION:
THE DECADE OF THE BRAIN

- *Jimmy calls himself "the walking wounded." He works as a messenger, delivering packages and letters to offices and apartments throughout downtown Orlando. He likes to wear a tie, even when the weather is hot and humid. He looks perfectly presentable; people who pass him occasionally smile hello. But if, say, a woman stopped and asked him for directions, Jimmy would first look at her blankly, then, he'd start to stammer. He might even get angry and spew out a string of obscenities. What this woman and others don't realize, at first, is that he had a severe head injury years ago. Jimmy's scars are invisible.*

- *Arlene was riding her brand-new bicycle down the hill near her house. She'd walked, run, ridden, and sledded down that hill so many times in her young life that she could close her eyes and instinctively know she had reached the bottom. That's exactly what she did this spring day. Unfortunately, she couldn't see the broken tree limb sitting in the middle of the road. She hit it at full speed, flew over the handle bars and hit her head. She is still in a rehabilitation hospital, recovering from her head injury.*

- *Sam loved his new position. As vice-president in charge of sales for a major corporation, his responsibilities were enormous. But, then again, Sam always did have a great deal of energy. He always had time to listen to his subordinates' complaints and suggestions. He met his deadlines and he was always one step ahead of the competition. In short, Sam was a one-man dynamo of executive capability, and it was no secret that he was being groomed for the corporation's top spot. But all this was before his accident. A two-car collision on the interstate left Sam befuddled, confused, and angry. Although he suffered only a mild*

1

*head injury, the damage was enough to sabotage his mana-
gerial talents. He could no longer lead—a fate Sam refused
to acknowledge. By not accepting this, Sam became an
unhappy, bitter alcoholic.*

These are only three short stories, three vignettes of
people whose lives have been irrevocably changed because
of a head injury. Unfortunately, they are not alone. Nor are
their accidents isolated ironies of life. A staggering 700,000
people suffer from traumatic brain damage every year, with
140,000 of them ultimately dying and between 70,000 and
90,000 permanently disabled. But there's more: *Only five
percent of them get the help they need.*

ONE LIFE TO LIVE

As late as the 1970s, 90 percent of all head-injured
patients died. Today, thanks to an abundance of medical
advances, higher-quality technology, and improved emergency care, more and more people are surviving—not only
Vietnam vets who sustained head injuries in battle, but
ordinary people with ordinary lives. Add the fact that
contemporary Americans take more risks—from skydiving
to mountain climbing, from driving cars at breakneck
speeds to pursuing the brass ring at any cost—and the
evidence is undeniably clear that head injury has indeed
become a "silent epidemic."

CAUSE AND EFFECT

It's a fact: A head injury can occur to anyone at any time.
But there are some specific arenas that put people more at
risk:
- *Men outnumber women two to one in head injuries—
  especially young men between the ages of 15 and 24.*
  Why? They are more apt to try something new, be it the
  "thrill" of a dare or a car race down a dark country lane.
  They also tend toward more physical—and more risky—
  work, such as hardhat, high-rise construction.
- *The young always take more "daredevil" chances*—with
  motorcycle, bicycle, and car crashes causing more head
  injuries than any other mode...
- *...but the figures climb back up again after the age of
  70,* with most head injuries the result of falls.

- *Bicycle accidents are becoming one of the major causes of head injury*—with over 1,300 deaths last year alone. But wearing a helmet can drastically cut down the risk.
- *The causes of head injury vary according to geography.* In our car-oriented San Antonio, Texas location, motor vehicles are the number-one culprit. In some cities, firearms and assaults account for most of the head injuries. In cities where there's a great deal of construction and development, industrial accidents cause the most damage.

MIND OVER MATTER

In many ways, the brain is our most vulnerable organ. An injury to the head doesn't heal the same way the heart, or the liver, or a broken leg does. It isn't a matter of "staying off your feet for a few weeks" or "getting plenty of rest" or "taking two aspirin and calling the doctor in the morning." Head injury affects who we are; the way we think, act, and feel. It can change everything about ourselves in a matter of seconds. And it can create havoc in the people we love, our family and friends, who are suddenly faced with a disabled stranger with:

- *Cognitive dysfunction*...including memory loss, perception and comprehension difficulties, and deficits in attention, organization, problem-solving skills, and reasoning.
- *Physical impairments*...including partial paralysis, spasticity, lack of coordination and balance, and swallowing difficulties.
- *Behavioral problems*...including over-aggressiveness, depression and mood swings, violence, and lack of impulse control.

But all is not bleak. The medical and technological advances that have kept head-injured patients alive have also developed better and more successful treatment.

THE "RE" FACTOR

Brain recovery often means extensive rehabilitation— retraining and relearning that requires time, consistency, expertise, and a structured, secure environment. In fact, *without* rehabilitation, the patient may stop far short of his potential. Here's proof: In a study of severely head-injured young adults with serious cognitive and emotional disturbances, 50 percent of those who received rehabilitation were found to be productive three-quarters of the time—as opposed to only 36 percent of those who did not receive treatment. Ultimately, they were not only less emotionally disturbed than those head-injured young adults who did not go through rehabilitation, but they also did better on memory and learning tests. Other studies of severely head-injured patients who had received rehabilitation found that many of them were able to become useful members of society—if they had a supportive atmosphere at work and at home.

These results are not surprising. It is only in a rehabilitation setting that a patient will have the most advanced equipment and most comprehensive care. And it is only in this setting that a family can get the education they desperately need to cope with the day-to-day problems that crop up in brain-injury—and to truly help their hurt loved ones.

But perhaps the most compelling reason for rehabilitation is its goal: independence. With successful treatment, a head-injured patient can regain at least some of his ability to:

1. Live, work, and enjoy life in our society.
2. Redevelop social and family relationships on a more equal basis.
3. Participate within the community.

However, proper rehabilitation doesn't come cheap. A person with a moderate head injury can conceivably spend more than $100,000 in treatment. The figure zooms literally into the millions for severely head-injured survivors who need between five and ten years of rehabilitation.

Fortunately, help is at hand. The U.S. government has recognized the fact that head injury is indeed a serious problem nationwide. Congress has declared the nineties "The Decade of the Brain," appropriating $15 million to the dual fields of head injury rehabilitation and head injury prevention.

The insurance industry, too, has discovered the benefits of rehabilitation in the bottom line: Every dollar used for head injury rehabilitation saves up to thirty-five dollars in future medical costs.

Yet, despite this important financial and public recognition, there is no denying the pain of the individual family, the individual victim—and the high cost of head injury in both emotional and practical terms. There is, after all, no price tag on loss, no "discounts" on the turnabout of fate. But there is hope.

And that's where this book comes in.

HEAD INJURY: A GUIDE FOR FAMILIES

Both of us have been involved in the field of head injury rehabilitation for many years. With our work at the Rehabilitation Institute of San Antonio (RIOSA) we have seen countless incapacitated head-injured patients become functioning members of society. Together, we have long felt the need for a clear and helpful guide for families who are thrust into the world of head injury, a book that would not only contain all necessary information, but offer reassurance as well. Thus, *Head Injury: A Guide for Families* was born, a book that not only addresses you, the family member, but medical professionals who are just now embarking on a career in head injury rehabilitation.

Within these pages, we will take you on a journey through the brain. You will discover how the brain works, and why. We will explore the many varied and complex symptoms that come into play when the head is injured. Step-by-step, we will show you the rehabilitation process—as well as offer sound advice on choosing the best rehabilitation hospital for your loved one. And, most important, we will pinpoint how you can help a head-injured survivor in the best and least stressful ways—for both of you.

Both of us know there is life after head injury. After reading this book, it is our hope that you, too, will believe this to be true.

ONE

AN ANATOMY LESSON

"What a piece of work is a man!"
—William Shakespeare
Hamlet, Act II, Scene 2

Picture this scenario: It is a bright summer day, a perfect Sunday in which you have nothing better to do than sleep, or think, or spend time with someone you love. As you prepare a picnic, you tuck in, amid the sandwiches and fruit, that new book you've been dying to read. You and your "significant other" drive out to the country, to an empty meadow. You lay out your blanket; you eat your food and talk of romance. Settling down, you lean back against the cool trunk of a spreading apple tree. You close your eyes; you feel the cool breeze on your flushed face. You sleep...and wake up with a start and an exclamation of pain. "Ow!" you say, rubbing your forehead. You look down by your leg and see the culprit: an overripe apple.

If your name was Newton, this situation might lead you to the discovery of gravity. But, if you are a mere mortal like the rest of us, you have just learned from an experience.

You have used your brain.

We are not often aware of our brain, of its unflinching attention throughout every second of our days—and nights. But think of it: In the above scenario, you anticipated a pleasant day. You organized and planned your picnic. You discussed love and life and felt the joy of real contentment. You ate your food; you swallowed your cider; you fell asleep. And, when your nap was interrupted, you perceived and understood how the apple fell from the tree. You learned not to go to sleep under any more apple trees. You stored this information and made it a part of your memory.... Yes, all these activities involve the brain—but they are only just a few examples of how your brain was involved, intertwined, and incorporated in your day!

The fact is, in many ways, the brain is a marvel. Although it weighs less than three pounds, it controls, initiates, stores, and comprehends every facet of our lives—from enabling us to automatically perform the proper steps for brushing our teeth to giving us the capability to feel the beauty and pathos of a concert symphony.

Under normal conditions, we don't give our brains another thought. We simply live our lives—until tragedy strikes. When a head injury occurs, the functions of the brain we take for granted can run amok. Depending on the location and severity of the injury, we feel its effects either cognitively, behaviorally, physically—or, more typically, as a combination of all three.

But unless you understand how a normal brain functions—how its different areas communicate with each other and with other parts of your body—you won't understand what happens when it is injured. Before you can discover what's wrong, you have to know what's right in....

THE ANATOMY OF THE BRAIN

Although it might look like a damp, frequently used sponge, don't let appearances fool you. The brain consists of a complex network of billions of nerve cells, called neurons. It has very specific locales, with each one responsible for a particular function. It can store tremendous amounts of information, and, when it is working properly, there is nothing in our manmade world that can compare to it—not even the most sophisticated computer.

The scarecrow in *The Wizard of Oz* bemoaned, "If I only had a brain." Well, if he did (and, as we all know, he only *thought* he didn't) it would be set up something like this:

1. The Peripheral Nervous System
Remember those Visible Man and Visible Woman dolls, the clear plastic ones with the veins and arteries all on display? Well, in the same way veins and arteries are intricately spread throughout the body, so are peripheral nerves. From the nerve endings at your fingertips to the nerves in your muscles, from the nerves entwined in your organs to the nerves attached to your spinal cord, all are in

play, all carry messages to the brain. The hot stove you touch, the ice-cold drink you taste, the tack under your bare foot—all these sensations, or stimuli, travel toward the brain to elicit a response. Then the brain sends a message back, and you quickly withdraw the sore foot. Without the brain's interpretation, the pain or the thirst-quenching feeling would be meaningless; you wouldn't feel or think anything of these sensations at all.

Think of the peripheral nervous system as a messenger service, traveling throughout the "city" of the body to pick up and deliver a specific action, thought, or sensation.

2. The CNS

No, it isn't a discount chain for men's fashion. CNS stands for the Central Nervous System or, to be more exact, the spinal cord and the brain. The CNS is the master control, the chief of all the nerves. The spinal cord is the first stop; it is a go-between, a relay station that connects the peripheral nervous system with the brain. Messages go up and down your spine, so to speak, delivering stimuli to the brain that must be interpreted, and then taking the brain's reply down to the rest of the body—either a response to speak, move, listen, gesture, show emotions, or any combination of these.

3. The Brainstem

Traveling up the spinal cord, we find the next stop on the "upper management floor": the brainstem. It consists of three areas:

Medulla, which is as basic as you can get. Here are the life-sustaining controls for blood pressure, heart rate, and breathing in and out.

Pons, which is a bridge linking the medulla to the higher, more evolved areas of the brain. Here, too, is the *recticular formation*. It is a conglomeration of nerve fibers, helping to control muscle tone, reflexes, wakefulness, and mechanisms to keep you alert and ready to react to change.

Midbrain, which gives you, and lower animals, eye muscle control and more "recticular formation" action—from staying more alert to keeping your reflexes honed. It is also a bridge between the brainstem and the cerebellum (see number 4, following).

The entire brain stem is attached to the spinal cord via thick nerve fibers.

4. The Cerebellum

Travel behind the brainstem, and you'll find the cerebellum, the area of the brain that regulates all your movements, balancing and adjusting every step and every stance. It's also a wonderful "traffic manager," smoothing and coordinating your movement and your speech muscles. *Basal ganglia*, located higher in the cerebrum (number 7, below), are its sidekicks, helping the cerebellum to modulate and modify all of your movements.

5. The Diencephalon

You'll find this area right above the brainstem and right below the majestic, higher-functioning cerebrum. It's the true gateway to higher thought and emotional depth—and not just because of its location. Why? Because it's home to the *hypothalamus* and the *thalamus*—two key players in the brain game.

All sensory information, from the ridiculous to the sublime, must first pass through the thalamus, which works like a switching station in a railroad yard. Here, your mother's meat loaf recipe will be delegated to your memory storage tank in the temporal lobe, at the same time the brainstem starts you salivating in anticipation of dinner. A Walt Whitman poem might find a place in your memory right next to the meatloaf, but its words also travel to the limbic system (number 6, following)—which controls your emotions. It might make you soar. Or, as the poem ricochets back and forth from the emotional limbic system to the more intellectual areas of the brain, you could find yourself contemplating the ironies of life.

In short, the thalamus is a beehive of activity, sorting out messages and deciding which areas of the brain get what.

As you might have guessed from its spelling, the hypothalamus is its cousin. No bigger than a pea, it rests right below the thalamus. But don't let its small size mislead you. The hypothalamus's influence is vast. From appetite control to sexual arousal, from thirst to sleep, from balancing body temperature to keeping hormonal secretion intact— the hypothalamus does all of these and more. And, because of its close proximity to the emotional limbic system and the intellectual cerebrum, it also plays a role in regulating your emotions, motivations, and moods.

6. The Limbic System

Anxiety. Joy. Anger. Elation. None of these emotions works in a vacuum. Thanks to the limbic system, the

HEADLINERS

A study printed in the *New England Journal of Medicine* proved, beyond a doubt, that bicycle helmets save lives. For one full year, Dr. Robert S. Thompson and his colleagues studied bicyclists who had sustained head injuries while bicycling. Their results? Ninety-nine cyclists had severe head injuries—*only 4 percent had been wearing helmets.* Those who wore helmets reduced their risk of head injury by a full 85 percent! Since most bicyclists are children, helmets can be considered a wise investment in everyone's future.

How to get your children to wear helmets? An evaluation of a community-wide helmet campaign in Seattle found that helmet wearing increased by 14 percent—but in Portland, where no such program existed, helmet use only increased from 1 percent to 3.6 percent. Get your schools, your communities, and your local government to act. Public campaigns work!

interlocking structures of nerve cells that run between the diencephalon and the intellectual cerebrum, you can literally feel and express your emotions. Because the limbic system lies so close to the cerebrum, your feelings are very much tied to your thoughts, perceptions, and attitudes. Without the Limbic System, you might cry or laugh—but it would signify nothing. With an intact Limbic System, you can have real emotion, filled with color and depth. You can feel the glory of that summer day in the apple orchard. You can feel embarrassed when the apple falls on your head. And because of the link between the limbic system and the intellectual cerebrum, you can remember this day not just as a series of events but as a look at the past.

7. *The Cerebrum*

This is the area of higher functioning thought, memory, and perception. As you might expect, this is the largest part of the brain—and it is home for several interrelated areas.

The *hippocampus* and the *amygdala* are responsible for emotion, memory, and thought. The hippocampus sits directly in the temporal lobe of the brain; it is connected to all your senses—and to the limbic system. Its sister, the amygdala, is nestled within the limbic system itself. Together, they can trigger a rush of emotions and coinciding thoughts. Let's go back to the apple orchard for an explanation:

It's now the cold of winter. You are hungry, but your refrigerator is bare except for some slowly rotting apples. You look at them; you smell their pungency. Thanks to the hippocampus, these senses connect you back to that summer day in the orchard, a memory that has been sitting in storage. These vivid memories now flooding the hippocampus trigger the limbic system into action. The system's amygdala comes to attention, rushing the flood of memory through the limbic network, flashing its own emotional images of that summer picnic into the nostalgic brew.

You remember. Your thoughts return to that day, and you can feel the emotion of the day.

The *cortex* is the gray lining that covers and clings to the cerebrum. Think of it as a stretchy, wrinkled blanket made of billions and billions of nerve cells that covers...

...the *cerebrum* itself, the chunky gray and white matter of the brain. Between the two lie all your thoughts, movements, and stored memories, all that you learn, understand, and communicate. Here is where you are most human—and most vulnerable when it comes to head injury.

The *corpus callosum* is similar, in many respects, to an interstate highway. Rich in nerve cells and fibers, it connects...

...the *right and left hemispheres* of the brain. Think of a line going down the middle of your brain, dividing it into two perfect mirror images—a right and a left side. Although pop psychologists have turned "right-brain" creative thought and "left-brain" logic into a magic formula to "find" the real you, in reality, both hemispheres work together, communicating via the corpus callosum. Here's an example of the right and left brain hemispheres in action:

You see somebody you'd like to know better. You approach him or her and start up a conversation. That's your left-brain in action. Perhaps you slowly drawl out your, "Hi." Perhaps you look right into the other person's eyes for dramatic effect. Or perhaps you make a joke, such as, "We have to stop meeting like this." Whatever "line" you choose, it's your left-brain that gives you the ability to speak and

LATERAL VIEW OF BRAIN

use language, but your right-brain gives what you say its dash of color.

Your left hemisphere is also more responsible for all your other language abilities—from reading to calculating and writing.

Your right side controls your visual memories, your ability to draw or copy, play music, or dance. It's also the right side that allows you to see the bigger picture, the consequences of your life further down the road.

When head injury occurs in only one hemisphere of the brain, the result is seen in the opposite side of the body. A damaged left brain could result in paralysis on the right side of the body, and vice versa. Emotional differences will also be noticed: Injury to the left hemisphere can commonly cause depression. But the same injury in the right hemisphere could actually make a person unaware of his deficits.

Not only is your brain divided in half, but each half has four lobes, each with a different function:

The *frontal lobes* are, of course, in front. They are, in many ways, the commanding officer of the brain. Here you will find controls for impulse, motivation, social abilities, expressive language, and voluntary movement; you'll also find the ability to retrieve memory from storage. These lobes also control your "executive functions"—which include the abilities to plan and organize, to stay focused, to make decisions, and set goals.

Unfortunately, the frontal lobes are very vulnerable to head injury. The traumatic results? She might not be able to say what she means. He might not be able to generate any new ideas. Her attention might be scattered. He might lose control over his impulses and become violent, abusive, and coarse.

The *temporal lobes* are just behind and below the frontal lobes; they are nestled above our ears. They are as vulnerable to head injury as frontal lobes. They hold the bulk of your memories, both recent and from the distant past. Here, too, is the home of the hippocampus and its bounty of emotional thoughts. The temporal lobes also control your ability to understand language and appreciate music. The temporal lobes are the processing house for your perceptions; they put "law and order" into incoming information, sequencing it, and making sense out of what you hear.

Damage to the temporal lobes can mean that she will have trouble remembering things she'd done just an hour ago. He might not be able to perceive what you mean. The Mozart she hears might sound like cacophony.

The *parietal lobes* sit above the ears, near the back of the brain. You might call these the "sensitive" lobes because they control your sense of touch, and they play a major role in your academic abilities, including reading comprehension and deciphering spatial relationships.

Damage here can hurt his ability to physically feel and recognize an object. She might find herself unable to read even simple sentences. He might find himself unable to distinguish an apple from an orange; to him, both appear equally strange.

The *occipital lobes* are literally "the eyes in the back of your head." They are responsible, purely and simply, for sight. If you injure your occipital lobes, you can become blind.

These, then, are the parts of the brain itself. But no man is an island—and no brain stands alone. In fact, it floats like Jell-O in what we call...

...*cerebrospinal fluid.* This is a clear liquid that surrounds the brain, nourishes it, and protects it much as an airbag might protect a passenger in a car. This fluid also fills the open spaces or ventricles of the brain. Six times a day, new fluid replaces the old.

The *cranium* is the skull that completely contains and protects the brain. But there's more to this floating, encased "cocoon"—and its lining of membranes—that, in his book, *Clinical Neuroanatomy Made Ridiculously Simple,* neurologist Dr. Stephen Goldberg calls "P.A.D." for short. In actuality, these membranes, or meninges, are:

1. The *pia*, a thin lining that literally hugs the brain.
2. The *arachnoid*, a spider-web-like lining that is sandwiched between the pia and...
3. The *dura*, which rests right up against the bone of the cranium. It is strong and durable.

The P.A.D., which surrounds the entire central nervous system, provides further protection for the brain. But when head injury occurs, the P.A.D., too, can be damaged, with blood hemorrhaging and collecting beneath or between the linings, severely complicating the initial injury.

Knowing the different areas of the brain and how they function is one thing, but understanding how they communicate with each other and with the rest of your body is another. Let's take a look at the message-relay system.

LINES OF COMMUNICATION

Remember your summer day in the orchard? The cool breeze, the delicious picnic, the pain when the apple fell on your head—all these facts had to be sent to your brain for decoding, deciphering, storing, and responding. Messages had to go back and forth throughout your brain, from your limbic system to your frontal lobe, from your right hemisphere to your left—not to mention the on-going, continuous messages for breathing in and out coming from your brainstem.

Scientists now know that these messages are conducted from nerve cell (neuron) to nerve cell via both electrical and chemical conductors. Fortunately, it's not as complicated as it sounds. Listen:

An electrical impulse carrying, say, the "ouch!" of pain from the falling apple, travels through a *neuron*, from its outlying *dendrite* tentacles to its central *cell body* and out again along a thin passageway called an *axon*. But as "ouch!" gets to the end of the axon, there's a space called a *synapse*. The next neuron lies in wait, but the electrical charge can't cross the synapse. "Ouch!" would become history at this point, except that the electrical impulse then triggers the release of a chemical, a *neurotransmitter*, which crosses the synapse to a *receptor* on the next cell. This starts the electrical conduction down the new axon. "Ouch!"

NERVE CELL, AXON AND SYNAPSE

continues on its way until it reaches a new synapse—where the electrochemical process once again takes place.

In fact, countless chemical neurotransmitters lie like silent wallflowers at the synapse, waiting for that one "Mr. or Ms. Right" to supply them with an electrical spark. In other words, only one specific electrical impulse will activate a specific neurotransmitter, and only one specific neurotransmitter will jump across the synapse and activate the electricity waiting in the new cell.

Now picture this activity occurring all over your brain at a fast and furious pace, relaying message after message to its different areas, deciphering, storing, and shouting commands all at the same time. Excuse the pun, but it boggles the mind how accurate, how attuned, and how precise the human brain remains, day after day!

From the need to yawn after your picnic lunch to the desire to sigh as the warm breeze hits your face, from the "ouch!" of the fallen apple to the "ah" of a kiss—the messages transported through your brain are as varied and unique as you are. But there is one basic theme to almost every chemical message that crosses over a synapse, as crucial a rule to remember as one plus one equals two:

HEADLINERS

"I evaluate myself in relationship to the way I was prior to the accident and in comparison to other victims. The characteristics of head injury vary from individual to individual, and the length of time since the injury is also a major factor. About three years ago, I did something very funny which was an example of the type of poor judgment encountered by head injury victims. I called the police to report a lost cereal bowl!

"Head trauma isn't like mumps or measles, which go away after you get them—it's with you for life. You just compensate for it. It's a long, rocky road. My lifetime goals are to excel as a father, a son, and as a husband. My accident didn't change these—it put an emphasis on them..."

—James Blakely, a head-injured person from Tucson, Arizona*

NEUROTRANSMITTERS CAN EITHER INHIBIT OR EXCITE ACTION, BUT MOST OF THEM INHIBIT

Yes, it's true. Most neurotransmitters soothe the savage beast. Left to your own devices, you might respond to "ouch!" with a grandslam throw of the apple in the vicinity of a nearby window—or your unlucky partner. You might further be inspired to add a few choice curses, followed by a temper tantrum in which you trampled the apple into mush.

Instead, the message you receive from your brain is, "Calm down," "stay cool," or even, "forget the apple. Go home, think about your day, and discover gravity."

Unfortunately, most of these inhibitory messages originate in the frontal lobes, which, as we have already mentioned, are especially prone to injury.

This is almost the end of the anatomy lesson. But there is one more rule to remember about the brain: the whole is

---

*Reprinted from "First Person Accounts" from the National Head Injury Foundation, Inc.

indeed much greater than its parts. Each of the various components, from the lobes to the hemispheres, from the neurotransmitters to the cerebrospinal fluid, work together to create... *you*—your unique personality, your unique attitudes, intelligence, and emotions. This "uniqueness" makes head injury all the more devastating when it occurs. By understanding how the normal brain functions, you will not only understand what happens when things go wrong, but you will be able to grasp how varied and individual the resulting symptoms can be.

Yet as singular as each case ultimately is, head injury happens in only a few basic ways. In fact, that's the subject of the very next chapter. Read on....

TWO

WHEN HEAD INJURY OCCURS

> "I used to think this kind of thing only happened on
> TV or in the newspaper—not to people I know and
> love. And especially not to me..."
> —A head-injured patient at RIOSA

Michael had always wanted to be an attorney. And at 35,
his dream had come true. He was a prominent attorney for
a top-notch Louisiana law firm. Michael worked hard—too
hard, if you asked his wife. When his old college buddy told
him about a great deal on a one-week fishing excursion in
Canada, even his wife urged him to go. He agreed. It was
time for a little R & R.

Unfortunately, it was rainy and windy their first two
days in the wilderness. The third day proved the same.
Impatient and suffering from cabin fever, Michael and his
buddy decided to go out on the lake anyway. But the
weather only got worse. Halfway across the water, the boat
began to pitch and roll. Michael fell and struck his head on
the side of the boat.

His friend managed to get him back to the cabin. Michael
had been unconscious for only 10 seconds, but he remained
dazed for five minutes more. He then complained that he
had a splitting headache; he felt dizzy and nauseous. But
his symptoms didn't seem that bad, and he didn't want to
spoil the trip—especially when the next day proved to be
sunny and warm.

Yet when he returned to the law firm, Michael still felt
dizzy and nauseous, and had an almost continuous headache. To add to his problems, he also found it difficult to
concentrate on his work. He couldn't look at a single file for

HEADLINERS

MIND MYTH # 1: If you've injured your head, doctors will identify it immediately.

Wrong. Head injuries can be "invisible." The amount of damage can't always be seen, even with a CT scan or a more advanced brain scanner called MRI (Magnetic Resonance Imaging.) Why?

• There are so many nerve fibers in the brain— billions and billions, actually—that it's difficult to pinpoint which are damaged and which are not.

• The damage, as in diffuse axonal injury, can be widespread—affecting many different areas of the brain.

• Microscopic damage can't always be picked up, by even the most advanced diagnostic tools. Yet microscopic damage can pack a wallop. It can cause problems such as depression and confusion, which are made worse when its victims are told "it's all in your head."

more than five or ten minutes; the words would start to blur together.

Michael decided his problems were caused by his eyes. He just needed new glasses, he thought. He went to his optometrist, who could find nothing wrong.

Michael's wife was getting upset. For the past few weeks, he had been acting peculiar. Formerly calm, caring, and stable, he had suddenly become a stranger. He was apathetic. He ignored the kids, and he had absolutely no interest in sex. He was easily frustrated and irritated. When the optometrist failed to find a problem, Michael's wife insisted he see their internist.

The internist referred Michael to a neurologist, who took a series of diagnostic X-ray tests that all proved negative. Later, however, Michael underwent neuropsychological testing that revealed that he had suffered a significant head injury, caused by his boating accident.

A rehabilitation program concentrating on attention and memory deficits helped Michael in only a few short months. Within three months, in fact, he was back on the job, a successful attorney who still worked too hard, but who made time for family vacations...on land.

It was several weeks before Michael's head injury was recognized for what it was—a situation that's more common than you might think. Head injury can be difficult to diagnose for several reasons:

• Its symptoms are easily labeled as something else—a case of flu, overwhelming stress, or, in Michael's case, the wrong eyeglass prescription.

• The resulting injury includes symptoms that are as individual as the victim himself.

• Not everyone who has an accident suffers from head injury. Another fisherman might have hit his head and suffered nothing more than a minor bump that went away within a day.

• Head injuries are sometimes so microscopic that, as with Michael, they are difficult to detect—even with the most advanced diagnostic tools. Yet small does not necessarily mean minor. Even the most microscopic brain injury can cause major problems.

Despite the masks that can conceal head injury from both patient and physician, certain universal characteristics act as clues.

HEADS UP

From strokes and tumors to Parkinson's Disease, your brain can be injured internally, without any outside intervention. But a discussion of these diseases belongs in a different book. The head injuries we're addressing here are the ones that are *traumatic*—that is, caused by a fall, or a car accident, or a bullet, or even a boat on a stormy lake. These injuries occur suddenly, without warning, interrupting what until then had been normal development.

A simple truth:

The brain governs and regulates everything that makes a person human—from the way he thinks to the way he acts, from the way he walks to the way he feels. Thus, damage to the brain may leave him significantly changed.

Like Michael, a calm person might suddenly become irritable at the slightest provocation. He might become self-destructive, reaching for drugs or alcohol to ease the pain. He might cry at the slightest provocation.

When you consider that damage may be contained in one specific area, creating very specific symptoms, or it may be widespread throughout the brain, creating many unpredictable symptoms—you get an idea of how complex a bump on the head can be.

SKULL DUGGERY

There's nothing like an imposing skull to send goosebumps down a horror fan's arms, but there's more to its shape than just the scare factor. Look again. It's completely smooth. But if you were to run your hands along its interior, you would notice "innards" that are rough, bony, and ridgy—especially the area near your forehead and ears where your frontal and temporal lobes reside. Under normal conditions, your brain is happily bobbing in its sea of cerebrospinal fluid. But if your head hit the steering wheel, if you fell off your motorcycle head-first without a helmet, if you slipped on a staircase and tumbled down twelve steps, your brain—along with the rest of your body—would get shook up. It would bounce and jiggle within its skull home, hitting and rehitting those bony ridges around your forehead. And which areas of the brain would most likely hit and rehit this ridgy skull zone? None other than the higher-functioning frontal and temporal lobes—which hold those thoughts, actions, and motivations that make you human and unique.

PUSH AND PULL

This starting-stopping movement of our brain when it is injured has a name. It's called an *acceleration-deceleration* injury.

Let's say you are driving along in your car (acceleration) until it crashes into a tree and comes to a sudden stop (deceleration). This abrupt acceleration-deceleration movement causes the brain to strike the bony ridges of the skull—resulting in bruising, hemorrhaging, and even stretching or tearing of the axons in the brain. The brain can also be bruised by a direct hit on the skull. Sometimes the impact causes the brain to move in the opposite direction, such that a blow to the front of the head causes a bruise in the back of the brain. This "backhand" phenomenon is called a *coup-contrecoup injury*.

HEADLINERS

MYELIN

Axons are covered with an insulation called myelin, which serves almost the same purpose as insulation on your electrical cords at home. This insulation protects the axons, and also helps conduct electricity at a much faster rate, sending those electrical messages we discussed in Chapter One at a fast clip. But when the axons are stretched, electricity cannot be conducted as quickly or efficiently. This *may* result in many of the physical, cognitive, and behavioral problems encountered in closed head injury. If the axon heals itself, all may eventually be well. But if the axon is severed or torn, it may not be able to repair itself—and the symptoms may be permanently disabling.

A COMMON FRONT

Most traumatic head injuries result from acceleration-deceleration action, and most of these head injuries result in frontal and temporal lobe bruising, which we call *fronto-temporal contusions*.

These bruises can create short- or long-term memory loss, as well as language deficiencies in either comprehension or production. Damage to these lobes can also affect motor skills and coordination, visual perception, attention, behavior and more—all symptoms that we will review in this book.

Adding insult to injury, there's more to brain damage than frontal-temporal contusion. In addition to the bouncing ball of the brain hitting the "concrete" wall of the skull, stretching and tearing can occur—with serious repercussions.

DIFFUSING THE ISSUE

The brain does not stand alone. As we mentioned in Chapter One, its stem is attached to the spinal cord via a cluster of thick nerve fibers. When the head is struck and the brain bounces back and forth, bounding and rebounding within the skull, these nerve fibers are pushed and pulled in all directions. In fact, when the head is hit with any sort of force and the brain is violently shaken, the nerve fibers (axons) within the brain can be stretched. A long, tumbling fall; a car crash that thrusts a victim through a shattered front window; a vicious fight—all these can cause widespread damage throughout the brain. Called *diffuse axonal injury*, this condition may result in a coma that can last anywhere from a few days to a few months...or years— especially when the brainstem nerve fibers are sheared. Because this area of the brain affects our very survival— from breathing to staying awake— damage here can be long-lasting and devastating.

A SWELLED HEAD

Unfortunately, head injury is a painful example of the whole that's greater than its parts. It's more than sheared nerve fibers and an acceleration-deceleration injury. A bruised brain can become swollen, the worse the damage, the more it will swell. Although that might not sound so serious in light of everything else we've discussed, *swelling is actually the major reason for brain damage.*

Think of it. When you bang your foot, say, against the coffee table, it will swell. Similarly, your brain will swell when hit. But there is a crucial difference: When your foot swells, it's easy enough not to go without shoes for a few days. But your brain is encased in a finite amount of space. When the brain swells, it has no room to expand within the confines of its rigid skull. Instead, *intracranial pressure* builds and builds, damaging even more nerves and causing even more pain.

It is crucial that the swelling be treated quickly. Unless medication and proper treatment to reduce the swelling are given in the acute-care hospital, the pressure will continue to build, damaging more and more nerves. (We'll discuss brain swelling and other secondary physical symptoms of head injury in more detail in Chapter Five.)

But wait. There's still more. Head injury is not only categorized as a possible fronto-temporal contusion, a diffuse axonal injury, or a swelling. It's also diagnosed according to whether the injury is open or closed....

AN OPEN BOOK

A bullet wound . . . a shard of glass . . . a forceful blow with a heavy instrument . . . any of these can penetrate the brain, damaging both it and its surrounding skull, causing both a skull fracture *and* brain injury. Any accident involving an outside force that penetrates the head is called an *open head injury*—which has its own problems, because:

- Pieces of skull, skin, hair, and debris are literally pushed into the brain, creating bruising, bleeding, and swelling. Add a skull fracture, and there is even more pressure on an already weakened brain.
- The foreign matter that has entered the brain makes infection a great risk.

CLOSED QUARTERS

Damage from a *closed head injury* is seemingly invisible. Because the skull is not penetrated, everything appears intact. But inside, the damage begins as the brain pounds against the bony ridges of the skull. Like Michael, who hit his head against the boat, some people with closed head injuries don't receive a proper diagnosis for several weeks or even months.

The majority of head injuries are closed. And a closed head injury is vulnerable to diffuse axonal injury and swelling. From memory loss to dizziness, there may be some sort of neurological impairment—sometimes temporary, but other times a permanent fact of life. . . .

You now know how the brain gets damaged. But that's still not enough. For physicians to diagnose the extent of a head injury, they must determine the *degree* of injury that has taken place. For them to create a helpful, constructive rehabilitation program—they must go beyond the diagnostic categories of open or closed, diffuse axonal injury, or frontal-temporal contusions. That's exactly what we'll discuss next.

THREE

DEGREES OF INJURY

> "Life is what happens while you are making other plans."
>
> —John Lennon (1940–1980)

MYTH: Someone with a mild head injury will always come out of it fine.
FACT: Not necessarily. Mild injury can hide microscopic damage, which can affect a person's thinking process, motor control, and mood.

MYTH: Someone who has had a severe brain injury will always be a "vegetable"—and would be better off dead.
FACT: Not so. Every day science offers new research and technology to help people live longer and better. We have seen victims of severe head injury progress from a deep, long-lasting coma to an ability to recognize loved ones, laugh, join a conversation—and contribute to society through work.

MYTH: No one ever gets better without rehabilitation.
FACT: Not always. Many people actually do have spontaneous recovery which occurs without rehabilitation care. However, a rehab hospital can provide a safe environment to prevent medical complications and provide social, physical, cognitive, and vocational skill training—all of which can help recovery flourish, spontaneously or not.

Perhaps it's because head injury involves the brain and the vast mysteries of the mind. Perhaps it's because the psyche is involved—the undefinable characteristics that make a person not only human, but unique. Perhaps it's because the injury occurs so swiftly, so traumatically—and

HEADLINERS

C IS FOR CONCUSSION

The word *concussion* is more confusing than you might think. On the one hand, a concussion is defined as a temporary loss of consciousness. But on the other hand, there doesn't have to be a loss of consciousness at all.

Further, one head injury predisposes a person to the cumulative effects of subsequent head injuries. A concussion might be the "ding" a third baseman hears for five to ten minutes after he's been hit by the ball, or the fumbling of a football quarterback who gets progressively worse after every tackle. The effects are cumulative—as for the "punch-drunk" fighter who can no longer hit a moving target or even see it. Brief episodes of memory loss may add up to periods of amnesia or permanent memory impairment.

can change life so irrevocably. Perhaps it's because so many areas of a person's being are affected—from the way he thinks to the way he walks across a room, from the way he conducts himself in public to the way he reads and writes. . . . Whatever the reasons, traumatic head injury is clouded with half-truths, myths, and erroneous beliefs.

This makes sense. Head injury is difficult to accept and to understand. It can be extremely complicated, involving so many diagnoses, so many treatments, so many symptoms.

But there's room for optimism.

CLASSIFIED INFORMATION

Despite the confusion, medical professionals and scientists have helped separate the wheat from the chaff. Categorizing the different ways that the brain can become injured helps doctors determine the severity of a head injury and predict what the outcome will be. Let's become familiar with these degrees of injury:

Classification # 1: Mild Head Injury

Seventy-five percent of all brain injuries are considered mild—the result of, say, a football tackle, a fall down some stairs, or a minor collision. Categorizing a head injury as mild means that:

1. The victim has been unconscious for less than twenty minutes—or he hasn't been unconscious at all.
2. He will have suffered some slight neurological impairment. Perhaps he's dizzy or nauseous. Perhaps his speech is slurred or his vision blurred. Whatever symptoms he may have, they will crop up within the first three months after the injury.
3. His hospital stay, if any, will usually last less than one week—just enough time for him to rest, to give his jolted, bruised, and banged-up brain a chance to heal, and to allow the physicians on staff to perform various diagnostic tests.

Sounds easy, right? Wrong. The word "mild" can be deceiving. Mild head injury can produce what's called *post-concussion syndrome*, which involves neurological and psychological problems. As we discussed in Chapter Two, microscopic damage is not always detected, even with the most advanced diagnostic tools. Although 50 percent of people suffering a mild head injury return to work or school within two weeks, *a significant one-third of victims are still unemployed three months down the road.*

In fact, mild head injury can lead to what medical professionals call *post-concussion syndrome*—which, if not recognized, can cause serious psychological and neurological damage. Here's how it works:

Joe is one of the best house painters around. But one particularly humid, hot day is getting to him. He can barely lift his arm; the smell of the paint is making him light-headed. He just wants to finish that last panel by the patio...almost done...a scream! Joe falls off his ladder onto the grass. He's dazed and unconscious. The homeowner, who ran outside when she heard Joe yell, immediately calls an ambulance. By the time it arrives ten minutes later, Joe is already awake. At the hospital, he's diagnosed as suffering from a mild head injury; his frontal-temporal contusions are so slight that they are not picked up by a CT scan or normal X-ray. After a few days, he's discharged from the hospital, ready to go back to work.

But over the next three months, neurological and psycho-

HEADLINERS

HEAD INJURY STATISTICS

- Most patients are young, single men between the ages of 16 and 25.
- The majority of injuries are the result of car accidents, but sports, the workplace, and assaults on the street also contribute their share.
- Alcohol intoxication plays a nasty role in head injury because it predisposes people to act recklessly—especially behind the wheel of a car. Drinking and driving should never mix, but too often they do.

---

logical difficulties develop. Joe becomes irritable. He can't remember simple things. He's restless, and he simply can't work on the task at hand. It takes forever to paint even the porch of one house. Unfortunately, his clients don't appreciate this. There's little sympathy. After all, they are paying Joe to paint their homes....

Fired from job after job, Joe becomes extremely depressed. He tries to get a job working as a painter for a large contractor, but he can only handle it for three weeks before he's fired once again. His depression spirals down, pushing his friends and his family further and further away. His wife starts to complain; Joe just isn't there anymore. He doesn't seem to care about the kids, and he gets so angry. Frankly, she's afraid.

Four months have now gone by. Joe's wife has left him, taking the kids. Joe is miserable. He has angry outbursts. There's only one thing that makes him feel better: alcohol. He starts to drink. He continues to drink. Soon, he does nothing but drink.

It isn't until a concerned friend gets him to enter an alcohol abuse program at a local hospital that Joe's problems are finally addressed. A neurologist on the hospital staff orders a series of neuropsychological tests, which reveal brain damage. At last Joe will receive the head injury rehabilitation treatment he so desperately needs....

Unfortunately, Joe lost a lot of valuable time. The sooner a person enters a program, the better the results. As Dr. Rebecca W. Rimel and her colleagues note in their article, "Characteristics of the Head Injured Patient" in *Rehabilita-*

tion of the Adult and Child with Traumatic Brain Injury:
"It should be remembered that often events occurring during the first hour after injury decide the eventual outcome for the patient. Therefore, rapid transfer of the head injured patient to the hospital is important, and a long period in which the patient is susceptible to additional insults to the nervous system should be avoided."

The exact figures aside, the main point to remember is that *time is of the essence in head injury.* Joe was in fact hospitalized after his fall from the ladder, but no one realized the extent of his brain injury. If someone had correctly diagnosed his continuing problems, and made sure he got proper rehabilitation as soon as possible, Joe would have avoided much anguish and pain. Now, he not only has to be treated for the neurological damage his injury caused, but also for depression and alcoholism.

Even more unfortunate than lack of quick detection is the fact that many doctors scoff off post-concussive syndrome as malingering—a way for a "needy" victim to get attention or compensation. Still others claim, "It's all in his head." In reality, as study after study has shown, post-concussive syndrome is likely to be a combination of both neurological and psychological problems. Incidentally, few of the head-injured patients we have treated have been malingerers. . . .

Classification # 2: Moderate Head Injury

This one's more serious. It means the person has been unconscious from one to twenty-four hours. It also means that he may be hospitalized for several weeks. Once the crisis has passed, he will probably be transferred to a rehabilitation hospital. The amount of time he will spend there will depend on the extent of his disabilities and on his progress, but it's likely he'll call the rehab hospital "home" for an extended period of time.

Symptoms vary from individual to individual, but moderate head-injured survivors may suffer from:

- Tremors or balance problems
- Weakness
- Paralysis
- Lack of coordination
- Seizures
- Language problems
- Memory deficits

- Perceptual difficulties
- Poor judgment and problem-solving
- Behavorial problems

More news: A study by Drs. D. W. Corthell and M. Tooman discovered that as many as two-thirds of survivors with a moderate head injury are unable to go back to work one year after the injury.

Classification # 3: Severe Head Injury

In severe head injury, brain damage will be deep and diffuse, and the victim will be in a coma for at least one day. He will have physical deficits; he probably will have muscle coordination problems, and he may be paralyzed or spastic. Rehabilitation is always required.

Severe head-injured survivors may go back to work after intensive vocational training, but usually in a reduced capacity. Many such victims must remain in the care of their family or a supported living environment.

Classification # 4: Catastrophic Head Injury

When physicians cite a "persistent vegetative state," they are usually referring to the consequence of catastrophic injuries. Here, victims will be in a deep coma for months, years, perhaps forever. They might have subtle sleep and wake cycles, but this is more of a "twilight" awareness, a barely conscious state of being alive. They must be fed; they cannot speak; they probably do not understand anything that is said to them. Unfortunately, even at the top rehabilitation hospitals these patients may fail to demonstrate improvement. However, an adequate trial of rehabilitation is in order before deciding on long-term placement.

This, then, is the medical "lingo" used to define the degrees of head injury. But, let's face it—when it's someone you love who's hurting, words, theories, and classifications mean less than: "Will he recover? Will the person I love be well again?"

For the answer to these hard questions, medical professionals use certain predictors of outcome. Although nothing is ever completely certain, although nothing is ever etched in stone, these predictors can at least offer clues to families and friends who desperately need to know.

In the next chapter, let's look at a doctor's detective work in action. . . .

HEADLINERS

It was a dream come true when 20-year-old Mark Giger met the National Honorary Chairperson of the National Head Injury Foundation—James Brady.

In 1987, Mark had been in a car crash. He was left in a coma that lasted almost three months—a severe head-injured young man.

According to an article in the NHIF Newsletter, "For Mark and his family, the months following his accident and his emergence from coma were filled with fears and frustrations. Mark often became depressed. It was during the early stages of his rehabilitation that his aunt saw Jim Brady speaking about the NHIF on a television talk show. Hoping that Jim would help her nephew, she called the White House . . ."

Although Mark's aunt didn't speak directly to James Brady, a message was given to him, and he wrote Mark a letter offering words of encouragement. "Keep fighting," he wrote. Mark has been fighting back ever since.

Although he has had to change his goals, Mark has been able to graduate with his class. He is enrolled as a day student in a local college. And, as the NHIF article concludes, "We think he's doing very well, indeed."

As adapted from a National Head Injury Foundation (NHIF) newsletter dated Winter 1989–90.

FOUR

THE DOCTOR AS DETECTIVE

Ned, a prominent TV personality, hated the idea of turning thirty. He knew that his looks and his health translated directly into success on the job. What Ned didn't know was that within a few short weeks, he'd be *hoping* to turn thirtysomething. It happened on a particularly sultry Los Angeles evening as he leaned against the railing of a second-floor apartment balcony, chatting with a woman he'd just met. Suddenly the railing gave way. Ned fell, struck his head on the concrete below, and lost consciousness.

This is what his acute-care hospital report said:

"In the emergency room he presented with a Glasgow Coma Scale of 8. CT scan revealed large blood clots over the surface of the left brain and a smaller one over the right side. There was a large bruise involving the right parietal region. The patient underwent approximately 13 hours of brain surgery and remained comatose and poorly responsive for two weeks. He started to awaken with poorly localized responses, only withdrawing an arm or leg to painful stimuli. He did not produce speech, nor did he show any recognition of voice. He subsequently made rapid physical improvement, being able to ambulate and speak. However, he had significant problems with confusion and disorientation...."

No, this is not shorthand medical lingo that only doctors with twenty years of experience could understand. What this report clearly presents in one brief paragraph is a head injury diagnosis. After you've read this chapter, you will understand the meaning of that diagnosis and others.

ONE, TWO, THREE, TESTING...

A study of patients undergoing head injury testing found that they were particularly likely to have *emotional distress* if their injury had occurred more than six months before and they had not received any help. These patients were apt to be anxious, depressed, confused, and socially withdrawn. The fact is that the sooner rehabilitation starts, the sooner the recovery process can begin. But before you can set up a treatment program, you need at least a preliminary diagnosis. And that starts with some basic diagnostic tools:

1. CT SCAN. Computerized Axial Tomography (CAT for short) has pretty much taken over the job plain x-rays used to do—especially for suspected head injuries. Although a CT scanner looks like something from a science-fiction movie, this large, donut-shaped machine is actually an x-ray camera that can take pictures of a person's brain in slices. Because it is able to photographically "peel away" layers of tissue, it can pinpoint problem areas—especially bruises and blood accumulation. A CT scan can help determine if surgery is needed.

CT scans are an especially good tool for exploring open head injury wounds. In fact, studies have found that CT scans have an almost 100 percent accuracy rate in identifying blood clots.

But nerve damage, which can be extremely subtle, may not be picked up in initial CT scans. Blood that seeps slowly from damaged tissues beneath the skull (called *subdural hematomas*) can also go unnoticed. Unfortunately, that means that the seeping blood has a chance to accumulate and put undue pressure on the brain, which leads to more nerve damage.

As you can see, more finely tuned diagnostic tools are needed. Luckily, such tools exist in today's world....

2. MRI. The newest "buzzword" in the diagnostic community, MRI, stands for *Magnetic Resonance Imaging.* Now for what it means: Combining physics and computer technology, MRIs are able to pinpoint problems that would never be seen on a CT scan. Like a highly evolved detector, an MRI uses radio frequencies and a magnet to chart the electrical charges created in the brain; it then converts them into computerized, highly detailed pictures of the brain. MRIs can display both focal and diffuse nerve damage.

But, when it comes to minor head injuries that cause

subtle cognitive damage, even the sophistication of an MRI might not be enough....

3. PET SCAN. A PET (*Positron Emission Tomography*) scan creates an actual map of the patient's brain. A tagged radioactive liquid is injected; as the liquid seeps throughout the brain, its movements are tracked and an individual portrait is created. PET scans have been found to show minor brain abnormalities that are not picked up by an MRI.

4. EEG. In electroencephalogram (EEG), electrodes attached to the scalp measure the electrical activity (waves) in the brain and show the results, either on graph paper or on a display screen. If someone has a moderate or severe head injury, chances are it will show up as an abnormal brain wave pattern or in an irregular brain wave speed.

5. Evoked Potentials. These are relatives of the EEG. Rather than passively measuring electrical activity, evoked potentials measure the brain's ability to *respond* to specific visual, auditory, and sensory stimuli. They help determine if the sensory pathways in the brain are damaged.

Other diagnostic tools you might hear mentioned include intracranial pressure monitoring, cerebral blood flow measurement, and measurements of cerebral metabolism.

THE ART OF PREDICTION

In addition to the tools created by modern technology, there are other useful predictors of outcome that have evolved through much research and scientific study. These low-tech predictors count on experienced doctors' ability to analyze and diagnose a head injury. The way the patient feels, reacts, and functions are key components in making a diagnosis. In medical detective work, the patient himself provides the most important clues of all.

Here's a brief description of these other tools that are used in rehabilitation hospitals nationwide:

Tool # 1: The Glasgow Coma Scale

Imagine a technique so simple that everyone, from the most highly trained neurologist to the newest nurse in the emergency ward, could use it to determine the severity of injury within those first crucial hours. This does in fact exist. It's the Glasgow Coma Scale, a universal system that rates the severity of a person's injury via his ability to open his eyes, move, and speak. The more severe the injury, the lower his performance, and the lower the number he is assigned. A very low number suggests very serious injury, and little likelihood of total recovery.

Here's a twist: severe injury doesn't always imply deep unconsciousness. It all has to do with the number on the scale. As far as gross observable changes go, the Glasgow Coma Scale works so well that it has only a 3 percent disagreement rate.

Here's what the scale looks like:

GLASGOW COMA SCALE*

Eye opening
Spontaneous..4
To speech 3
To pain...2
None...1
Best motor response
Obeys commands..6
Moves within the general locale..5
Withdraws...4
Abnormal muscle bending and flexing...................................3
Involuntary muscle straightening and extending...............2
None...1
Verbal response
Is oriented..5
Confused conversation 4
Inappropriate words..3
Incomprehensible sounds..2
None...1

But as good a common denominator as it is, the Glasgow Coma Scale does have its limitations. Yes, it does its job of predicting early outcome—and it certainly helps determine whether someone will live or die. But the scale can only measure neurological deficits; it cannot predict how someone will eventually function in the outside world and it does not predict independence.

Other predictors of outcome are needed....

---

*Adapted from *Pediatric Head Trauma: A Guide for Families* by Ann V. Deaton, Ph.D., Healthcare International, 1987.

Tool # 2: Post-Traumatic Amnesia (PTA)

As you can probably guess, this predictor has to do with memory. In fact, it's a useful guide to determine cognitive outcome within the first year.

Here's how it *doesn't* work:

When a head-injured patient wakes up from a coma, he doesn't sit upright and cheerfully ask for the person he loves. Nor does he ask for some good, hot food, as actors are prone to do on prime-time soaps.

Here's how it *does* work:

Waking up from a coma is an extremely gradual process, and the part of the conscious mind that takes the *longest* to recover is memory. The loss of remembering day-to-day events after injury is so prevalent, in fact, that it has a name: *Post-Traumatic* Amnesia.

PTA is categorized from the moment of the accident to the time when a patient becomes lucid, remembering day-to-day events in a continuous memory. The longer the memory loss after the accident, the more serious the injury—and the less the chances for a good recovery.

In the interim, before their memory clicks in, head-injured patients may not understand where they are—or even *who* they are. Some patients become extremely agitated and cannot be comforted. When their memory comes back, they usually have little or no recollection of their hours, days, or months of post-traumatic amnesia time.

As a rule, a patient who has PTA for less than one hour is diagnosed as having a mild head injury. One to twenty-four hours translates into moderate head injury. Anything longer than twenty-four hours is considered severe. This is an important reality for families to face, because they usually feel absolutely joyous when their loved one awakens from a coma after "only" four days. *But* if both the Glasgow Coma Scale and PTA point to severe head injury, the patient will most likely have long-term cognitive and behavioral deficits.

PTA as a predictor tool is not absolute. It's difficult to pinpoint its time line exactly. Not only is the patient confused, but family members or significant others are usually too overwhelmed to recall accurately when their loved one began to remember. Then, too, as a patient regains consciousness he'll be inconsistent, remembering the time one day but not the next, recalling your name at five o'clock but not at six. This makes it hard to use the PTA as a predictor of outcome.

Thus, other tests are *still* needed. . . .

HEADLINERS

YOU MUST REMEMBER THIS

We know families that keep trying and trying to get their head-injured loved one to remember the accident that started it all. They'll coach their loved one as if the World Series were at stake, or at least the college boards. But in fact, the majority of head-injured survivors *never* remember their accident. This has nothing whatsoever to do with their ability to recover. Call it ironic. Call it fascinating. But also, call it normal.

Tool # 3: The Rancho Los Amigos Scale of Cognitive Functioning

Developed at California's Rancho Los Amigos Hospital, this scale is divided into eight stages, with a gradual progression from deep coma to appropriate behavior and cognitive functioning.

Why use the Rancho Los Amigos Scale? It's a quick, handy universal shorthand to diagnose and communicate a patient's level of functioning. It also can be used to guide and develop individual rehabilitation programs. Here's a brief description of its eight stages:

Level I: No Response. The patient is unconscious. He appears to be sleeping. He does not respond to any stimuli presented to him. This comatose state can last for seconds, minutes, hours, days, weeks—or even months.

Level II: Generalized Response. Here, the patient will react—but inconsistently and without purpose. His response, often a gross body movement or a garbled vocalization, is usually the same—regardless of what Glasgow stimulus is used. But his first response is activated, more times than not, from deep pain.

Level III: Localized Response. The patient is improving. He will react more specifically to different stimuli, but his response will be inconsistent. For example, he may occasionally turn his head in the direction of a speaker's voice. He may have a vague awareness of his body. He may inconsistently follow simple commands such as "close your eyes" or "squeeze my hand."

Level IV: Confused—Agitated. The patient has become very active, but he is not yet able to understand what's going on. His behavior might become bizarre; he might cry out or try to remove his feeding tube. He may be hostile and uncooperative, but he is not acting out of malice. It's a reaction to his overwhelming confusion.

Level V: Confused—Inappropriate. The patient has become less agitated; he will respond to simple commands in a more consistent manner. But if the commands are more complex, he gets confused and gives random, incorrect responses. He may become agitated if he is in a noisy or "busy" environment. He will not take the initiative. He will respond best to his body's aches and pains, to his own comfort, and to close family members. His memory is severely impaired, and he is unable to learn new information. At this level, he is in danger of "wandering off" the ward.

Level VI: Confused—Appropriate. Things are looking up. The patient is motivated, but still depends on others to lead the way toward his goals. His reactions will be more appropriate. If he is uncomfortable he will complain. He is beginning to recognize therapy staff members, and is much more aware of himself and his family. He can easily follow simple directions. His memory of the past has improved greatly, but his memory of recent events is still impaired.

Level VII: Automatic—Appropriate. The patient seems to act appropriately in the hospital and at home. He is now oriented to person, place, and time in these settings. All seems well—but things are still not completely right. He goes through his daily routines automatically, like a robot. Although he can dress, wash and feed himself independently, he needs supervision to ensure his safety. His judgment and problem-solving skills are still impaired, and he cannot make realistic plans for his future.

Level VIII: Purposeful and Appropriate. At last! The patient can integrate the past with recent events. He is independent and functional in society. However, he may have subtle difficulties with reasoning, judgment, and processing information—especially in high stress, unusual, or emergency situations. He may be actively involved in a vocational rehabilitation program, learning a new way to live in his new world.

This hierarchy of levels looks simple and straightforward. But in real life, not every head-injured survivor moves smoothly through each level. A patient may move from Level II to Level IV and never demonstrate any true Level III behaviors. Or, a patient may reach Level III and never progress beyond that point. Even if your loved one reaches Level VIII, it won't necessarily mean he is exactly as he once was. As mentioned earlier, he will, most likely, be changed—in ways that are subtle or not so subtle. To determine these "finely tuned" changes, medical professionals must turn to other means....

Tool # 4: Neuropsychological Testing

Written questionnaires. Mazes. Blocks. Storybooks. These are some of the tools of the neuropsychological testing trade. Varied and carefully plotted, these tests can help determine within eight to ten hours what the previous diagnostic techniques may not:

- *Behavioral problems*, such as the capacity for violent outbursts or immature behavior
- *Emotional problems*, such as depression, anxiety, or distress
- *Cognitive problems*, such as sequencing difficulties or attention deficits

These tests can also help a rehabilitation team separate those dysfunctions caused by accident-related neurological damage from those with a psychological base. For example, memory complaints might be the result of temporal lobe damage and difficulty sustaining attention—or an emotional response to overwhelming stress and depression. Anxiety and depression can make it difficult to concentrate and attend to tasks. A person who's nervous tends to be forgetful.

Neuropsychological testing can also help identify a patient's primary problem and isolate it from any secondary problems it might have caused. Another example: Let's say a head-injured person has trouble both comprehending what he reads and following instructions. However, tests performed by the rehabilitation team may show that these are only *secondary* problems caused by a primary problem: inability to pay attention. Tackle the attention deficit, and

---

HEADLINERS

Here is a dialogue that took place during a neuro-psychological testing session with a "very pleasant, mildly retarded teenager" with central nervous system problems, a young man who was becoming overwhelmed by the tests:

*"He leaned across the table, smiled at the examiner, patted her hand very gently, and making a fist with his other hand, shook it and rather regretfully said, 'I'm going to have to hit you.' The examiner said, 'This is kind of hard, isn't it James?' James looked very relieved and said, 'Yes!' "

---

chances are the patient's comprehension and ability to follow directions will improve. Without outside distraction or with repetition he may be able to concentrate on what he's reading—and enjoy it more. Without the benefit of test results as a guide, a rehabilitation therapist might try everything in the book to improve a patient's reading comprehension—to no avail. Until the patient improves his attention skills, the other problems may never go away.

Some of the neuropsychological tests include:

• *Serial addition test.* In this test the patient is asked to listen to numbers and add them together sequentially. For example, he will hear three plus five and state "eight." Then he will hear the number five and should respond "thirteen." This is a sensitive test of memory skills.

• *Tactual performance test.* Here, the patient is blindfolded and seated at a table holding a board and 10 wooden blocks. He must replace all the blocks without looking, using first his dominant hand, then his non–dominant hand. He's then instructed to take off his blindfold and draw the board and the blocks from memory. Motor skills, problem-solving, spatial and tactile memory, and learning ability can all be analyzed with this one simple test.

---

*Excerpted from: "Cognitive, Personality, and Psychosocial Factors in the Neuropsychological Assessment of Brain-Injured Patients" by George P. Prigatano, Mary Pepping, and Pamela Klonoff from *Clinical Neuropsychology of Intervention*. Norwell, Mass.: Martinus Nijhoff Publishing, 1986.

• *Finger tapping test.* Using a mechanical counter or a metronome, the patient taps in rhythm as rapidly as possible for 10 seconds, using both his dominant and non—dominant hands. This test will tell a rehabilitation team if a patient has possible cerebellar dysfunction or problems with motor speed.

• *Family Assessment Device (FAD).* This 60-item questionnaire is given to family members to determine how well they function together as a family unit, to what degree they are capable of helping their head-injured loved one, and whether they themselves have any psychological problems that might have predisposed the patient to injury.

There's a real need for neuropsychological testing; it's an excellent tool that will tell you the specific cognitive and behavioral skills that need work. The tests have a 74 to 90 percent accuracy rate, but *proper interpretation is crucial*: they are only as good as the person administering them. A sensitive clinician must determine whether a patient's . . .

• Anxiety is an ongoing concern—or simply pre-testing jitters.
• Behavioral problems were in place well before the injury.
• Primary and secondary problems are hidden by the unique, highly focused, one-on-one testing environment. A patient might be at his best in the testing room—but only because he's the focus of one person's complete attention for hours.
• Test results can also pinpoint secondary psychological problems. Immaturity, selfishness, rudeness, depression—all can come out not only during the testing procedure, but during break-time conversation.

Tool # 5: Pre-injury Characteristics

Research has suggested that head injury may not always strike entirely at random. Learning-disabled children, impulsive and aggressive young adults, alcohol- and drug-abusing adolescents—all are predisposed to injury. In fact, one particular study of head-injured patients with a pre-injury history of drug abuse discovered that they had *twice* as many behavioral problems as patients who had never abused drugs. The behavioral problems didn't surface until late in the recovery process—frustrating family members and hospital staff alike.

The family circle also plays a role. Families with a head-injured member have been found to have more depres-

---

HEADLINERS

Here are some questions from a Patient Competency Rating Form* used at Presbyterian Hospital in Oklahoma City. Patients are asked to rate themselves either as *"Can't do," "Can do with some difficulty,"* or *Can do with ease:"*

How much of a problem do I have in...

1. ...preparing my own meals?
2. ...dressing myself?
3. ...remembering names of people I see often?
4. ...driving a car if I have to?
5. ...controlling crying?
6. ...recognizing when something I say or do has upset someone else?
7. ...controlling my temper when something upsets me?

This same form is also given to family members to see whether their observations and perceptions are the same—or whether the patient or a family member is denying certain problems.

---

sion, more instability, and more social disadvantages than other families.

Here are several pre-injury traits that predict a favorable outcome:

• *A "fighter" personality.* Someone who had been strong before her accident, who was patient, who was motivated and achievement-oriented, stands a good chance of regaining these traits and getting through the rehabilitation process with success.

• *Youth.* Studies have found that fewer children die from head injuries than their adult counterparts. In fact, the younger the person, the better the chances of successful

---

*Questions excerpted from Prigatano, George P. and Others. *Neuropsychological Rehabilitation after Brain Injury.* The Johns Hopkins University Press, Baltimore/London, 1985, p. 63.

rehabilitation. (The reasons involve the flexibility or "plasticity" of a child's brain—which we'll discuss later.)

• *Intelligence*. The smarter the person, the more likely he will benefit from rehabilitation techniques.

• *Self-control*. If a head-injured person has been able to retain (or re-master) his self-control, he'll also be better able to control inappropriate behavior and impulsiveness— possibly re-entering the community much sooner than his out-of-control, undisciplined counterpart.

• *Strong family ties*. The more love, support, and encouragement the patient feels from his family, the more it will help his rehabilitation—and his future care. In fact, the role of the family is so crucial an issue in head-injury rehabilitation that we give the subject its own chapter.

• *Similarity of pre-injury career skills and post-injury skills*. If a head-injured person had a fairly uncomplicated job, he'll probably have an easier time re-entering the job market than someone who is, say, a lawyer—whose organizational and memory problems will prevent him from exercising his profession.

• *Good coping skills*. Someone who knew how to relax and handle stress before her injury will cope better with the stress and trauma associated with head injury.

• *Solid financial support*. It's a fact of life: Rehabilitation hospitals are expensive. In order to receive the best possible care, patients need either good financial resources or adequate health insurance. Unfortunately, the majority of head-injury patients don't get help because they don't have adequate coverage—and they don't know where to turn. If only they were aware of all the potential sources of aid! Good rehabilitation hospitals have case managers or social workers to help families find the money they need—either through government funding or private foundations.

• *Deficit-awareness*. More than anything else, a head-injured patient must become aware of his problems. Even the most reputable and sophisticated rehabilitation program will not work if a person is unaware of his deficits. Deficit-awareness is *crucial*. A person must ultimately recognize his new limitations if he's to actively participate and return to his community.

As time marches on, these pre-injury characteristics become more and more important as diagnostic tools. A patient's personality, his lifestyle, his coping skills, his home or hospital environment—all these play a major role in predicting ultimate success.

Before we close the file on this particular piece of detective work, it's important to remember that predictions can be wrong. Diagnostic tools, research, and scientific studies can only show us so much. We cannot tell which of the billions of brain cells are dead—and which are merely damaged. We cannot tell if or when a person will suddenly have some spontaneous recovery. We cannot tell with any certainty which patient will plateau and never get beyond, say Rancho Los Amigos Level Five.

Recovery takes time. The symptoms that appear after a head injury can linger for a long while. They can even create more symptoms, with a life of their own. To cope with this confusing time, you should understand what the possible symptoms are—and why they may exist in your head-injured loved one. Let's go on to these symptoms now. . . .

FIVE

PHYSICAL SYMPTOMS OF HEAD INJURY

"I used to jog four miles a day to stay in shape. Now I get to have my own personal trainer. I have a physical therapist who works on my legs...They won't move."
—A former high school soccer star at RIOSA

Susan loved to feel the wind in her hair. In fact, that was one of the main reasons she loved to ride her bicycle. Eight years ago, when the city had had a transportation strike, getting to and from work became everyone's biggest problem. Susan got out her old rusty three-speeder. Within the first half-mile down the avenue, she'd regained her balance, her speed—and her love for bike riding.

The years went by. The strike was long over, but Susan continued to ride her bike wherever she went. She began to take weekend biking trips in the country. Some of the people she met on her trips wore helmets, but Susan thought that was being overly cautious. She referred to the helmets as "the new Yuppie toy."

Unfortunately, Susan didn't have the last laugh. On her ride out of the city one Friday night, she hit a pothole that she never even saw. She was flung over the handlebars, and hit her head on the concrete street.

By the time the ambulance brought her to the nearest hospital, Susan had already regained consciousness. But she was confused; she couldn't remember what had happened. A CT scan showed some bruising in her frontal and temporal lobes and a large blood clot in her brain. The brain had swelled, and intracranial pressure was building. Susan was rushed into surgery. After four hours on the operating table, she was put in intensive care and watched around the clock, receiving medication to reduce the swelling further and to prevent seizures. Eventually she was referred to a rehabilitation hospital.

Susan was alive and awake; she remembered who and where she was. Her parents were grateful that they had their daughter back. Her friends and co-workers were relieved. None of them—not even Susan herself—knew how close Susan had come to death—not because of her initial fall, but because of the secondary physical problems the head injury caused.

Before being tested for any neurological or psychological problems, before tackling any cognitive retraining, a head-injured person literally has to fight for her life. One life-threatening result of her injury may be hematoma.

HEMATOMA

When the brain is bruised, it may bleed. The more it bleeds, the more it will swell—and the larger the accumulation of blood. The act of bleeding is called *hemorrhage* and the collection of blood is called a *hematoma*. Now, when this pool of blood actually fills up *within* the brain, it's known as an *intracerebral hematoma*. When the blood is collecting between the brain and the dura (which, as described in Chapter One, is a durable membrane that covers the brain), it's called a *subdural hematoma*.

It might not be easy to stop a bleeding hand or leg, but at least the bleeding is visible. When the brain bleeds, it's all internal; nothing can be seen. And, as you saw in Chapter Four, even the most sophisticated diagnostic tools don't always pick up a deadly bruise.

But there's more:

The more the brain is damaged, the greater the risk of secondary swelling and bleeding.

Unfortunately, as we explained earlier, swelling and bleeding go hand-in-hand to create a dangerous buildup of pressure, which can damage even more brain cells than the initial head injury did.

What happens to this swollen brain? Unless the intracranial pressure is relieved via medication or surgery, the ever-expanding brain will find space only by pushing and squeezing down on the brainstem, the all-important area of the brain that regulates vital functions—from heartbeat to breathing.

Think of it: The heartbeat slows. The breath is barely audible. Biochemical and mechanical functions of the brain go haywire, leading to widespread damage throughout the entire body. The brain's blood flow trickles down to nothing. The brain no longer receives the bloodstream's life-giving oxygen, resulting in hypoxia. Ultimately, more brain cells die, causing brain tissue death.

Susan was lucky. She was injured in a large city, where she was taken to a hospital quickly and received the care she needed. Her brain swelling (or *edema*) was brought down; damage was minimal. After rehabilitation, she returned to her city life and her job as a dental technician, and led virtually the same life as before—with one crucial difference. She got herself the best bike helmet money could buy.

PHYSICAL EDUCATION

Secondary medical problems that can result from a head injury are only part of the story. The physical symptoms or deficits that the injury causes tells another tale. Let's examine some of these symptoms now:

Seizures

In ancient times, epilepsy was considered a curse from the gods—for understandable reasons. When epilepsy occurs as a result of head injury it can occasionally cause further injury. Any seizure starts with a burst of abnormal electrical activity somewhere in the brain. Seizures come in several different types:

Generalized or *grand mal* seizures are full-blown, involving widespread muscle contractions, rapid body movements, loss of bladder and bowel control, irregular breathing, and loss of consciousness. There is usually no warning. However, some patients do know when they are going to have a seizure; we call this feeling an aura. A common aura is a full feeling in the pit of the stomach that moves up toward the mouth.

Partial or *focal* seizures are a more subtle variety. Here, the head-injured person merely has a total lapse of concentration. She might lose the thread of what she was doing, or stop talking in mid-sentence, or perform a repetitive task such as picking at her clothes. Partial seizures, which frequently arise from the temporal lobe, may be difficult to diagnose. A common form is called complex partial seizures. Focal seizures may involve jerking movements of only one arm or leg, without loss of consciousness.

Seizures occur in 35 percent of patients with open head injuries. Although most seizures occur within the first week after an injury, the first one may not occur until one to two *years* following the head injury. Regardless of the time lag, the technical term for seizure following a head injury is posttraumatic epilepsy.

Seizures are unpredictable. A patient may not be considered free of symptoms until two or three seizure-free years have passed. Even then, there is a 5 percent chance that another seizure will occur down the road. Epilepsy needs to be carefully monitored by a physician who is familiar with the correct use of antiseizure medications.

The good news is that only 1 percent of "closed" head injury patients develop seizures. Therefore, most of these patients do not need to be placed on medication.

Loss of Motor Control and Coordination

A head-injured survivor in a wheelchair, learning to use it on different terrains...A right-handed man with *hemiplegia* (paralysis of either the right or left side of the body), learning to write with his left hand...A woman with *ataxia*, an awkward, unbalanced, and uncoordinated way of walking...A former athlete whose muscle strength and endurance is weakened, relearning to lift weights...A woman who appears frozen in time, her joints rigid and set in a beckoning pose...An adult man lying curled up in a fetal position, immobile...A knitter who can no longer hold her knitting needles, whose fingers have lost their agility and dexterity...A man whose motions are quick and brisk, quivering in spasticity...Physical impairments such as these are much easier to detect than cognitive or behavioral deficits, because they involve the parts of the brain that control what we can observe at a glance: body movement, muscle tone, and balance.

You may recall reading or hearing that the left side of the brain controls the right side of the body, and vice-versa. A head-injury survivor with a blood clot or contusion on one side of the brain may have paralysis of the opposite side of the body; this is called hemiparesis or hemiplegia. Paralysis is commonly more severe in the arm than in the leg. As time passes, it's possible that the person will regain the ability to move his arm, but still won't be able to manage finely coordinated movements such as buttoning a shirt or manipulating coins. Therapists will help him work on increasing his strength and compensating for those lost muscle functions.

Walking difficulty, called ataxia, may respond to physical therapy and medications, but is often very difficult to treat. It's frustrating when the person has enough physical strength to walk, but lacks the necessary sense of balance. Such a person usually needs to adapt to using a wheelchair.

Spasticity, which is abnormally increased muscle tone frequently seen in paralyzed arms and legs, interferes with movement and can also be painful. It frequently improves in response to changes in position, and also to stretching exercises. (A stretching routine, incidentally, is very important for almost all head-injury survivors).

Medications, including Lioresal (baclofen), Dantrium (dantrolene sodium), and Valium (diazepam), can be useful in treating spasticity. However, these medications are a mixed blessing because they may also cause weakness and sedation. If a patient needs all his available muscle tone in order to walk, the medication that relieves his spasticity may actually prevent him from walking. Thus, the doctor who prescribes the medication must carefully consider the relative weight of benefits versus side effects.

Sensory Problems

Our sensory perceptions are a product of both cognitive and physical abilities. We need to have the capability to understand, analyze, and remember in order to recognize and process what we see, hear, touch, taste, and smell. But we also need the ability to sense something in the first place. We need to *physically* see, hear, touch, taste, or smell. Unfortunately, this physical ability may be lost with head injury. Damage to the occipital lobe can cause blindness. Sometimes *diplopia*, or double vision, occurs as a result of cranial nerve damage or muscle imbalance. The visual fields can become constricted, due to injury within the visual pathways to the higher-functioning portions of the brain.

Sensitivity in the mouth can change as a result of head injury. Hot foods can seem so hot they can't be swallowed. Cold foods can seem much too frigid. And sometimes taste is totally lost, as well as the ability to hear sounds or feel objects.

Head injury frequently damages the nerves that carry

the sense of smell: the person may be left with a faulty
"sniffer" or none at all. Unfortunately, this type of damage
rarely improves with time, since it stems from permanent
destruction of the cells that respond to smells.

Sometimes a head-injured survivor is perfectly able to
see and feel, say, a hairbrush, but has lost her ability to
process the sensory input. Perhaps when she looks at the
hairbrush she sees a toothbrush and puts it in her mouth.
This is called a perceptual problem.

Sometimes the person recovering from a head injury is
perfectly capable of moving his arm or leg, but has a severe
handicap because he can no longer keep track of where it is
in space: he has suffered *proprioception* damage. To appreciate the function of proprioception, close your eyes and then
touch the tip of your nose. You knew just how to move your
arm and hand, didn't you? That's because your proprioception
was intact. To rehabilitation professionals, patients with
proprioception difficulties present a major challenge.

Speaking and Swallowing Disorders

A person doesn't normally give her mouth too much
thought, unless she's brushing her teeth, for instance, or
putting on lipstick. But her oral muscle function may
become severely limited if head injury damages a cranial
nerve. She may have a hard time articulating the words
she wants to say, because the muscles needed to produce
speech have become weak or have lost their coordination.
This condition, called *dysarthria*, may cause her speech to
be extremely slurred, or slower or quieter than normal,
making it hard for others to understand her. A person
whose head injury has damaged her ability to chew and
swallow efficiently is said to have *dysphagia*. If the dysphagia is so severe that it results in malnutrition, or causes
her to have a chronic problem with food falling into her
airway, she may need to receive all her nutrition through a
feeding tube.

Fatigue and Headaches

Fatigue and headaches affect nearly everyone at one time
or another. Unfortunately, it's not simply a matter of "take
two aspirin and call in the morning" when head injury is
involved. Fatigue and head pain can interfere with rehabilitation, requiring breaks that will slow down the process—
and possibly create future problems.

HEADLINERS

ALCOHOL AND HEAD INJURY DON'T MIX

A study of 102 head-injury survivors admitted to a trauma center found that those who had been under the influence of alcohol at the time of admission were:

- more agitated—for a long period of time
- discharged with lower cognitive abilities
- more neurologically and behaviorally affected by their injury
- more apt to ultimately die at a young age

In addition, people who have been head-injured have a *lowered tolerance* for alcohol. Depression, physical limitations, and the lack of access to quality long-term care makes many head-injury survivors turn to alcohol as a way to cope with their problems. Of course, alcohol ultimately, makes their problems even worse.

It's important not to exercise to the point of fatigue, and to devise a realistic schedule that includes rest periods. Inadequate rest can lead to increased agitation, behavior difficulties, and decreased attention.

Headaches are common following head injury, but do not signify new or increasing brain injury. Headaches tend to be more of a problem following mild head injury. Most headaches can be successfully treated with the same medications that are used for migraine headaches.

Bladder and Bowel Incontinence

No, this doesn't just happen in old age. Loss of bladder and bowel control is a very real—and very unnerving—physical disability. It's also tied into cognitive awareness. Remember when you toilet-trained your child? It took time, patience, and self-knowledge. All this can fall apart when a person sustains a head injury. The head injured survivor may have difficulty urinating, requiring intermittent catheterization (placing a tube in the bladder). Or she may suffer a loss of bladder control (incontinence). Incontinence can be treated by offering her the opportunity to go to the bathroom every two hours. Occasionally formal bladder tests (urodynamics) are needed to identify the problem clearly. Most people with bladder trouble can be kept dry through medication, catheterization, and timed voiding. Likewise, timed bowel programs can prevent embarrassing mishaps. Constipation, which is common among people who are physically inactive, frequently responds to increasing intakes of fluid, fiber, and fruit. Bowel stimulants, stool softeners, and bulking agents can relieve constipation for most people.

As difficult as some of these physical impairments seem, they are actually the easiest ones to accept and rehabilitate. In fact, a study by Dr. Yehuda Ben-Yishay found that over 80 percent of head-injured patients had an excellent physical recovery by the end of one year. The more lasting problems came from cognitive and behavioral deficits. These were the ones that determined a patient's ultimate social and personal adjustment—his or her ability to function once again in society.

It's easier to cope with someone in a wheelchair than someone who hurls abuse at every turn. It's also more accepted. The physically handicapped are finally getting the recognition they need and deserve—from access ramps to braille-numbered elevators, from closed captions to convenient parking spaces.

Unfortunately, head injury also causes invisible symptoms. Perhaps you sat next to one of the "walking wounded" when you rode the train to work this morning. Or, closer to home, perhaps your head-injured husband just doesn't laugh the way he used to, in that carefree way that made you fall in love with him. Worse yet, what if he doesn't remember getting married to you—or even what your name is?

An employer typically has less patience than a spouse or family member for these "walking wounded" head-injury survivors. A C.E.O. will proudly cut the ribbon to inaugurate the company's new offices built with access ramps for the handicapped. He'll have his picture taken with his first employee in a wheelchair. But he'll find it hard to justify paying someone who throws typewriters against the wall, can't meet deadlines, and refuses to get along with co-workers.

In short, physical problems are difficult, but cognitive and behavioral deficits can be an even greater handicap. Learning what the cognitive and behavioral symptoms are will help you cope—and help the person you love get better. Let's move on to examine these "invisible," yet very noticeable, effects of head injury. . . .

SIX

COGNITIVE SYMPTOMS OF HEAD INJURY

"I think, therefore I am."

—Rene Descartes

Lorraine had always been a top–notch secretary. In fact, her firm voted her Secretary of the Year six years in a row. But then Lorraine was in an accident; a car driven by a drunk driver smashed into her car's rear end. She lost consciousness for almost half an hour. When she came to in the emergency room, she was confused. She couldn't remember what had happened. The diagnosis? Lorraine had a closed head injury, with damage to her frontal and temporal lobes. Later, after three weeks at an acute-care hospital, she was admitted to a rehabilitation hospital.

While Lorraine was recuperating, everyone at work sent flowers. Her boss visited her once a week; her friends called at least once every other day. Within a month, Lorraine appeared to have regained her memory. She progressed rapidly, and after six months she was speaking and walking on her own. She could read, attend to her daily hygiene, and, all in all, seemed independent and ready to get on with her life.

The day Lorraine returned to the office, the entire staff threw her a party. There were strawberries and champagne, a three-layered cake, and a leather attaché case as a gift. Lorraine was exhilarated. She'd never felt happier in her life; she'd never appreciated life more. She couldn't wait to get back to her desk and begin working again.

That first week, all went well. Lorraine was the embodiment of confidence. She came into her boss's office, steno pad in hand, efficient and raring to go every time her boss buzzed. Lorraine told the boss not to worry—she would handle that MacGregor account herself. She would also do some research into that company they were thinking of buying. Lorraine said she planned on staying late the next few days so that she could refile all the notes on that Smith & Stein debacle.

But two weeks went by, and Lorraine's boss had only signed about four letters. She had yet to see the research on the new firm, and MacGregor was calling her twice a day now about his account. She didn't know what to do. She cared about Lorraine, but the work wasn't getting done.

Something had to be done. One evening, after Lorraine had bid her good-night, the boss sat down at Lorraine's desk. She had never snooped before, but she had to see for herself what was going on.

She was shocked. Lorraine's steno pads were filled with pencil sketches of flowers and random words in flowing script. Work to be filed was stashed away in a drawer. The files themselves were a mess, unalphabetized and overflowing. There were no notations on MacGregor, the new firm, anything else for that matter. Just dirty coffee cups, drawings, and empty Cheeto bags. . . .

When the boss confronted her the next day, Lorraine was aghast. She couldn't understand what the problem was. She had said she'd handle the MacGregor account—she just needed a little time. She would be happy to type up some letters, but she had misplaced her steno pad. And as far as the new firm was concerned, she had been about to make some calls when she was buzzed to come in. Why was her boss giving her such a hard time?

Clearly something was wrong. Lorraine was defensive. Both she and her boss knew she wasn't doing her work, but neither one knew why. They hadn't a clue. Her boss had no choice but to let her go. She gave Lorraine a decent severance package, but Lorraine was heartsick. She just needed time, that's all. She shouldn't have been fired; there wasn't enough cause. She tried to rally her co-workers against her boss; she wanted to sue the firm.

It all came to naught, however, because the Secretary of the Year could no longer handle the responsibilities of the job. Unfortunately, it had nothing to do with a sudden "mental breakdown." It had everything to do with Lorraine's head injury seven months before.

Lorraine's story is only one out of thousands of incidents

HEADLINERS

"Looking back on this entire incident, I realize that it was the most significant and influential event of my life. As a thirteen-year-old, I had never stopped to examine everything I had. I had simply taken for granted my health, my life, and, more importantly, the lives of each member of my family. It was this incredible realization of mortality which struck me the hardest. I was surrounded by friends and relatives but I cannot remember a more intense feeling of being isolated and alone. It had taken a tragedy such as this to enable me to fully appreciate my own life...

"Of course, there were times when even my parents broke down under the tremendous pressure they felt. I remember sitting in the hospital dayroom with my father, my mother, my brother, and my sister, sobbing, thinking only of what Lenny meant to us. He was physically as close as the intensive care unit next door, but too far away from us to make contact with him. We all shared the same feeling of helplessness, and I believe it was this that brought us so close together as a family. We became open and honest in our communication with each other. Our conversations included all the positive memories of our growing up years. We supported each other with hope and encouragement. We cried together; we laughed together; we prayed together. Most important of all, we needed each other."

—"Reflections of a Brother," by Michael Burke*

that occur each year. More than anything else, cognitive deficits mean a change of life.

KNOWLEDGE IS POWER

Cognitive meant "to know" in ancient Greek. Today, it means our intellectual, information-processing abilities.

---

*Reprinted from "First Person Accounts" from the National Head Injury Foundation, Inc.

Performance, attention, organization, planning, memory, flexibility, perception, and sensitivity all come under the cognitive umbrella. Unfortunately, these intellectual functions are concentrated in our frontal and temporal lobes—which, as we have seen, usually get the thrust of a fall, an accident, or a traumatic assault.

Knowledge is power—and the root of its power is understanding. Before you can cope with a loved one's cognitive deficits, you must understand what they are. Before you can help a loved one regain his cognitive abilities, you have to know what is possible—and what is not. Based on the classifications delineated by neuropsychologist George P. Prigatano, here are some aspects of cognition that may be faulty in a cognitively disabled person:

Mindset # 1: Attention and Concentration

A driver doesn't see the light change from red to green at an intersection. A student is too busy listening to the "boom box" radio outside his classroom window to finish writing an essay on a test. A guest at a party stops in midsentence and abruptly begins talking about something else. These are all examples of attention and concentration deficits that may be daily occurrences for the head-injured.

Think of it: Without the ability to pay attention, a person can't work productively or even stay involved in a conversation in a social setting. In fact, the functions of attention and concentration are both prerequisites for any higher mental task. They set the scene for independent living, career advancement, and even social relationships.

Other complaints that go along with attention and concentration deficits are fatigue, an increased need for sleep, easy distractibility, an inability to shift from topic to topic while engaged in conversation, and a lack of focus.

Mindset # 2: Initiation and Planning of Goal-Directed Activities

Interview any executive and you will hear him or her spout long-range plans, solutions to budgetary problems, and ways to implement better attitudes and health among employees. Whether or not you agree with the proposals, the fact remains that the executive can reel them off. This is a facet of what is aptly called executive function—the ability to plan, initiate, direct and monitor one's activities. But many brain-injured people have *impaired executive function.* Like Lorraine in the example at the beginning of this chapter, they frequently miss the point. They lack the "building-block" cognitive skills needed to perform executive functions. In addition to the attention and concentration difficulties discussed earlier:

• *They may have difficulty understanding the abstract.* In other words, they're only able to take things literally. For example, George, a head-injured teen, got into his friend Paul's car. Paul told him to put on his belt. George looked at him incredulously. "I already have my belt, on. Look." And he pointed to his waist where, indeed, he had a brown leather belt buckled around his pants. George didn't understand that Paul meant his *seat* belt.

• *Often, they can't stop talking or performing a task once they start.* A person with this particular deficit will ask the same question over and over again, making social interaction almost impossible. She might discuss a topic that had been dropped a long time before. He might continue vacuuming the living room carpet for hours—until someone says, "Stop!"

• *They may have difficulty solving problems in a realistic way.* Here's an example: Mike, a head-injured teen, decided that he wanted to go to college in the fall, but he couldn't take the necessary steps to put his plan in action. Rather than checking a college directory, sending away for bulletins, and applying to a few schools, he drove out to a nearby college on the first day of classes and asked where he should put his bags. Sally, a head-injured adolescent in her senior year of high school, let the whole first semester slip away while she stared out her bedroom window, ready and willing to tell anyone who listened that she was going to college . . . soon.

• *They have difficulty keeping the steps of a task in order.* This is called a sequencing deficit. She might take a dustpan out to the garbage before sweeping the floor. He might dry the dirty pots before they are washed—if he initiates any action in the first place. Usually, head-injured people with impairment of executive functions have difficulty initiating actions unless they're specifically asked or cued.

Mildly head-injured people with impairment of executive functions may be unaware that anything is wrong. They blame the misplaced work, the overdue deadline, the long

---

HEADLINERS
ATTENTION PLEASE!

There are two types of attention:

• *Sustained* attention gives you the ability to concentrate on one specific task, conversation, movie, or TV show for a specific amount of time.

• *Selective* attention allows you to focus on one thing while lots of other things are going on around you. A student can listen to a teacher's lecture while "tuning out" the sound of the lawn mower outside the window. A beer-bellied husband can watch the football game on TV while "tuning out" his mother-in-law's small talk. An executive can listen to a sales pitch over lunch while "tuning out" the sounds of the other diners.

---

absences, on others. That's because they have poor deficit awareness—that is, a lack of understanding about their disability.

• *They have trouble learning from their mistakes—and their successes.* You might say this is true for all of us at one time or another, but a head-injured person with this cognitive deficit might, say, continue to knock on his boss's door after it had been slammed in his face. Or a head-injured teen might receive a special dessert from her mother if she had cleaned up her room—but when her mother tells her that this is a reward for a task well done, the teenager gives her a puzzled look.

Impairment of executive functions might be a common deficit, but it's not an easy one to accept. One study found that 90 percent of head-injured people suffering from impairment of executive function could not handle vocational training.

Mindset # 3: Judgment and Perception

This mindset gets to the very heart of thinking. Without the ability to judge or perceive a situation, a person cannot analyze it. She will have trouble interpreting the actions or the intentions of others. He will be confused when he gets more than one piece of information at a time. She will "talk a good game," but there will be nothing behind her words. He will have an unrealistic appraisal of himself, of his strengths and weaknesses. She won't be able to correct or monitor her behavior. In short, life and its struggles, its joys and its tragedies, becomes devoid of meaning for anything deeper than an after-dinner sweet....

Here are two examples: Joe thinks he is the hottest thing in town—despite the fact that he's really thirty pounds overweight and in need of a shave and a job. Alice, on the other hand, has trouble with the larger picture. When her boyfriend got sick, she kept whining that he wasn't paying enough attention to her. Soon her whining turned to anger.

These two examples also point out an outgrowth of this mindset: denial. Judgment and perception are not just necessary qualities to view the outside world—they are also necessary for self-awareness. If you can't accurately perceive or judge your situation, you'll never realize that you have a problem. One of our patients at RIOSA was a prominent New Jersey lawyer and amateur pilot. He had been in a car crash and suffered a mild head injury. Most of the damage was in the frontal areas of his brain, which lead to impairment of executive function. He could no longer practice law. Unfortunately, he didn't believe he had any problems. He went back to his law firm ·and was subsequently asked to "retire." More dangerously, he tried to go up in his two-seater plane—and fly solo.

Self-awareness is the ultimate function—for everyone. Teaching a head-injured person that he is indeed disabled, and that he now has judgment and perception impairments, is a prerequisite for successful rehabilitation. We'll discuss some of the ways we teach self-awareness at RIOSA later on in the book.

Mindset # 4: Learning and Memory

Memory problems are thought to be the result of temporal lobe damage (where most memory is stored) or damage to the hippocampus (which is responsible for registering and retrieving information). In one study, 86 percent of severely memory-impaired head-injury patients had hippocampal damage.

Naturally a lack of memory will hinder rehabilitation—and re-entry into the community. In a different study, 65 percent of head-injured persons who could not find work had memory impairment.

HEADLINERS

SEEING IS BELIEVING?

Even if a head-injured person's five senses are intact, his problems with perception will also create sensory impairments. His hearing might be fine, but if he can't perceive that the car honking outside is waiting for him to put on his coat and leave, it doesn't much matter that he can hear every honk. He might have 20/20 vision, but if he can't perceive that the hornet he sees flying near him is going to sting him, seeing, quite literally, isn't believing.

Memory also reflects the other mindsets. It's simple: If you cannot perceive something, you can't learn it. If you can't learn it, you can't remember it.

Here are some examples of very real problems that memory deficits create, as excerpted from *Life After Head Injury: Who Am I?* by The Tampa General Rehabilitation Center.*

1. You are attempting to give directions to a friend, but you're not able to recall the names of the streets or the number of your new apartment.
2. You are about to help your spouse with the bills and have misplaced all the bills and the checkbook.
3. You call all women you know by "Hey, you!" or "Hey, doll!" simply because you are not able to remember their names.
4. You fail to improve any of your work skills, and you're passed over for a promotion, because you can't remember how to perform aspects of your job that are new since you came back after your accident.
5. You are completely confused when someone asks you a question about a meeting the two of you had last week. You do not recall the meeting.

Unfortunately, memory problems are very stubborn. Even when patients in a rehabilitation hospital were asked to

---

*Published by HDI Publishers in Houston, Texas, 1989. Reprinted by permission.

repeat the hour of their therapy appointment (which was at the same time every day), it took between four and eight weeks for them to memorize this one simple fact.

Because memory is so intricately involved in day-to-day living, memory problems are among the most important to overcome. In Chapter Ten, we'll discuss some of the rehabilitation techniques that are used to "jog" a head-injured person's memory.

Mindset # 5: Speed of Information Processing

When the brainstem is injured, it can create a "slow-motion" effect. Simple tasks can take forever. A patient might remember what his name is and can even write it down—if you give him ten minutes. She'll say good-bye to you—after you've already hung up the phone.

Unfortunately, speed is of the essence in our society. Families are quick to lose their patience when dealing with this deficit. It can be extremely frustrating to wait many seconds for a loved one to respond to the simple question, "What did you do today?" When there's no immediate response, the family member may repeat the question. Still no response. While the head-injured survivor is taking time to process the question, and struggling to remember the day's events, the other person may get irritated, thinking to herself, "He just isn't listening to me." She may compound the problem by asking a different question before he has had time to respond to the first.

Mindset # 6: Communication

All of us have times when it is just too hard to communicate what we want to get across. This can be an ongoing problem for the head-injured. Their language and communication problems usually stem from damage to the left hemisphere of the brain.

Here are some examples:

She might have trouble naming an object. She knows that the door has just opened, but she cannot seem to say the word "door."

He might have difficulty remembering the word he wants to use; it will always be "on the tip of my tongue."

She might slur her words.

He might speak too slowly.

She might have had an incredible vocabulary before her car accident, one befitting the English teacher she was.

But that was before. She now has a vocabulary of twenty words.

He might talk without thinking first. Lacking an inhibiting "social censor," he'll tell the woman sitting next to him on the bus that she's "as fat as a pig." He'll tell his boss that he doesn't feel like typing any letters right now—or ever again, for that matter.

She might talk too much, without letting another person get a word in edgewise. These last two examples involve behavioral abnormalities that affect communication.

Communication is not just the power of speech. It's also the ability to comprehend language and to express one's thoughts and ideas—all of which can be hindered in a head injury. The result is a "wandering mind." For example, Julie started discussing her new ad campaign with her client—only to begin talking, without skipping a beat, about the traffic en route to the city that morning. Unfortunately, the client didn't know that Julie had suffered a mild head injury. He just found her odd, rude, and irritating. And he hated the campaign.

Language disorders can involve both spoken and written words. In the same way that a novice student of French may understand much of the spoken language without being able to speak it well himself, so a head-injured person might be able to follow what you say to him but be unable to respond appropriately. Also, he might comprehend what he reads but not be capable of writing his thoughts down on paper.

These, then, are the mindsets that interfere with a person's ability to function on the job, at home—and in society at large. And, as if it weren't enough that a person can't remember a recent fact, that she can't write her name, that he can no longer think logically, cognitive problems also create *behavioral problems*. That's what we'll be looking at next.

Frustration. Irritation. Depression. Disinhibition. All these can have cognitive roots; all may be the result of brain damage. All have far-reaching consequences for a head-injured person and for those who love him or her. Read on. . . .

SEVEN

BEHAVIORAL SYMPTOMS OF HEAD INJURY

"I can't help it, but sometimes I gotta wonder, 'Why me?'"

—A 28-year-old former plant manager, a patient at RIOSA

• Sally was a real clothes horse before her head injury. She had so many outfits, shoes, and accessories that she had to have a consultant come in and help her design an organized, space-saving closet. But now she changes her clothes every single time she walks into her room—throwing the slinky black dress she wore for breakfast onto the ever-growing pile on the floor, and rifling through her closet for a ski jacket to wear for lunch.

• Milton never had a weight problem before his head injury. He loved a good steak and fries as much as the next guy but he worked it off in his company's gym. And, unless he was out celebrating, he only ate when he was hungry. But now he's like a speeding train, shoveling down food before it has a chance to cool on his plate. Day and night, you'll find Milton at the kitchen table or a TV table—eating anything and everything in sight.

• Since Savannah returned home from the rehabilitation hospital, she's been improving by leaps and bounds. She's never late for her therapy appointments. She eats her meals at specific times. She works hard at keeping up her personal grooming habits. But there is one problem

Savannah's mother didn't discover—until the damage was done. It seemed Savannah loved the catalogs that came in the mail. She'd think nothing of picking up the phone and ordering whatever she wanted. T-shirts, a vacuum cleaner, a china pet bowl, silk flowers—you name it and Savannah charged it by phone. When the items came to the house, Savannah didn't want them any more. Nor did she have the money to pay for them.

• George was a model husband and father before his head injury. Conservative and upright to the core, he was considered the quintessential family man. But lately upper management has been getting some disturbing reports. George pinched several of the secretaries as they walked down the corridor. He made lewd remarks at the last sales presentation. He made a pass at a colleague. He was sexually out of control.

• Timothy was always the class clown. Ever since fifth grade, he had been a mobile comedy act. Even the teachers couldn't help but laugh at some of his antics. But after he fell off his bicycle, Timothy changed; his jokes became nasty. He told one teacher she was disgusting and fat. He told a friend that he was the biggest nerd walking on two feet. He snipped off a girl's long ponytail. And to make matters worse, he didn't shut up. All day long he talked. During class. During assemblies. During the walk to school. Soon Timothy was talking only to himself. None of his old friends would go near him. And his teachers were losing their patience.

Different ages. Different lives. Different people with one common link: all of them were victims of head injury. And all of them are suffering because of inappropriate behavior they can't control—or understand.

AN ACT IS AN ACT IS AN ACT

Human beings function at higher levels than their animal counterparts. The fact is that we can think. We can plan long-term goals. We can formulate strategy. We can put ideas into action. But there's even something beyond "cognitive awareness." We humans can also *feel*.

Feelings at their most rudimentary level are common to all the higher species. Take one brainstem, some basic

HEADLINERS

MYTH: PROBLEM BEHAVIOR IN THE HEAD-INJURED GETS BETTER WITH TIME

Unfortunately, it's usually the other way around. A 1983 study of relatives of head-injured patients revealed that during the first six months after the injury, the relatives noted a minimal amount of psychological problems such as depression, irritability, or anger. During the second six months, however, there was an *increase* in these psychological problems. It was within this time period that most patients tried to adjust to normal life. They tried to re-enter the community or the work force, and found that they were not welcome. They also became aware of their new limitations. During the third six-month period, many of these same patients had withdrawn socially; they chose isolation rather than try to overcome the negative aspects of their environment.

Another study interviewed the families of head-injured patients at yearly intervals. The results? At one year, they felt their loved one had undergone significant personality changes. They were more excitable, more irritable—or completely unemotional. At two years, their loved ones were still irritable, but now they were also inclined to act out in socially inappropriate ways. After five years, these families were still citing behavioral problems as the worst result of their loved one's accident.

sensory perception equipment, and decent motor function—and any animal, from a snake to a squirrel, will feel pain or contentment.

But these are feelings without perspective. Only humans can *interpret* their feelings. And only humans have the cognitive ability to control their emotions. A woman who has just broken up with her fiancé is in tears, but she must muster her self-control, because she has an important business meeting in half an hour. A man is furious when a taxi driver slams into his car. He gets out, ready to fight—until he sees that the taxi driver is over six feet tall and built like Arnold Schwarzenegger.

These are only two small examples, but they show that cognitive abilities and emotions are closely aligned. Just as cognitive functions are vulnerable to head injury, so are the emotions—and the ways they make people behave. In fact, there are three facets to the behavioral symptoms of head injury—three "hats" that can play havoc with emotions, behavior, and life in the world at large:

HAT # 1: Neurological Damage

In Chapter One, you learned how most neurotransmitters in the brain *inhibit* behavior. When the delicate balance of neurotransmitters is disrupted, they can no longer do their job. Your emotional balance gets upset; you may suddenly say things that formerly you might only have thought, or you might act with the emotional immaturity of a young child.

Unfortunately, most of the inhibiting neurotransmitters inhabit the frontal and temporal lobes—which, as you now know, are often damaged in a head injury.

One reason behavioral problems rear their head is that head injured survivors no longer have the cognitive skills to perceive, understand, plan, or communicate appropriately. Without an apparatus for logic, Sally, the clothes horse, won't know that she shouldn't wear an evening gown to breakfast. Without a perceptive social censor, George doesn't realize that his sexual advances are inappropriate. Without the ability to recognize that he is full (or the memory that he has just eaten), Milton can consume food at an astounding rate. Here's another head injury fact:

Damaged or deficient neurotransmitters combined with a lack of cognitive skills translates into inappropriate behavior.

But neurological damage is only one-third of the story.

HAT # 2: Reactionary Disturbances

When a head-injured person first awakens from a coma, he may be agitated and confused. Think about it. Here he is in a strange hospital room, lying in a strange bed—without a clue as to how he got there or, in some cases, who he is.

Later, as he becomes more oriented, his agitation will turn to general irritability—which can last for days, months, or, in some cases, until the day he dies. This irritability comes from frustration; he can't do the simple tasks he'd always done before. Writing a check becomes a long, involved chore. Going to the supermarket is so complicated that it is impossible. Driving the kids to school can never be done again; he can't remember where the school is....

Sometimes irritability goes hand-in-hand with denial. As we have seen in Chapter Five, denial can have a neurological base (*anosognosia*). But denial can also have a life of its own—as a psychological reaction to the injury. A patient might become defensive whenever his limitations are pointed out. He might get belligerent when he discovers that his old goals are impossible to achieve. He might refuse to acknowledge his impairments, becoming angry and withdrawn when he can't do something. In full-blown denial, a patient will protect his old sense of self at any cost, making rehabilitation almost impossible.

In time, most patients do come to terms with their new limitations. Unfortunately, this new awareness can trigger yet another type of reaction. Without proper rehabilitation and good outside support, it sometimes becomes the springboard for drug and alcohol abuse, withdrawal, or even suicide.

Of course, we're talking about *depression*. Though it's sometimes the product of a chemical imbalance, depression can also be a reaction to a new and frightening reality. A patient might feel incompetent and worthless, hopeless and helpless. Occasionally these negative feelings so overwhelm a head-injured patient that nothing can help; nothing can break through the pain. Dr. Kurt Goldstein called this aura of complete and utter despair a *catastrophic reaction*.

Fortunately, most head-injured survivors have a milder form of depression, but it is painful nonetheless. Some of the signs are:

• *Psychosomatic pain.* He complains about the ache in his leg, the pounding in his brain, but there is no evidence of anything physically wrong.

• *A general loss of self-esteem.* When she realizes that she cannot organize her thoughts the way she once did, she feels less of a person. She hates the way she looks, the way she talks, even the way she now holds a knife and fork.

• *Mood swings.* One moment he'll be crying at a welcome-home party; the next, he'll be screaming at his wife for cooking a dish he hates.

• *Anxiety.* She is filled with nervous tension. She can't help it. Ever since she became aware of her limitations, she has been afraid—of people laughing at the way she speaks, of dressing wrong, of being unemployed, of not being able to handle a purchase at the five & dime, of being alone, unloved, and unwanted....

• *Sleep disturbances.* A study by Dr. George Prigatano et al discovered that head-injured survivors woke up more during the night, and had fewer deep sleep cycles, than their healthy counterparts. This lack of balanced, rhythmic sleep can create more depression—as well as irritability and anxiety.

• *Suicidal thoughts.* A study of depressed head-injured World War II soldiers found that the risk of suicide was still present 15 to 20 years after the injury. The possibility always exists. Listen to your head-injured loved one. Watch him. At the first sign of danger, contact your physician.

Head injury is a devastating trauma. The way a person reacts to it will be no less dramatic. The loss of your friends, of your place in the family sphere, of your career, your wishes and aspirations, of that person you once were and knew so well—all these cause strong emotional reactions: anger, depression, irritability, and more. And because there are usually cognitive deficits at work as well, these reactions will usually appear in disruptive, socially inappropriate—and sometimes dangerous—ways.

HAT # 3: Pre-Existing Conditions

In a strange way, head-injured survivors sometimes become more of what they were. For example, someone who abused alcohol or drugs before his head injury will probably try to cope with his new limitations in the same way. One particular study of head-injured patients who had a prior history of substance abuse or sexual promiscuity discovered that in most cases the injury, far from improving the situation, actually *amplified* pre-existing problems.

For example, Margo, a pretty 20-year-old single woman, suffered a mild head injury in a car accident. After months of rehabilitation, she was sent back home to live with her frail, elderly parents. Almost at once, Margo began to act in socially inappropriate ways. She began to dress provocatively; she wore a great deal of makeup; she spent much of her time out of the house. Her parents were worried sick;

they had no idea how to handle her. But when Margo's social worker questioned them, they admitted that Margo had *always* been promiscuous. She was acting the way she always had—but more dramatically.

Whether they're the result of neurological damage, a reaction to an unfriendly world, or a magnification of pre-existing conditions, behavioral symptoms are hard to take—for everyone. But forewarned is forearmed. You now know something of the general symptoms of depression, agitation, and irritability. In order to better recognize other, more specific signs of inappropriate behavior, read on:

1. "Get Out of My Room!" or Verbal Outbursts

Verbal outbursts are unpleasant—especially if you're on the receiving end. They explode, as if out of nowhere, but the patient soon forgets them. Verbal outbursts stem from a faulty limbic system—the area of the brain responsible for emotional states—and can occur sporadically throughout the head-injured survivor's life.

Oddly enough, these verbal outbursts rarely take place after major crises. Rather, the patient will lash out at the minor, insignificant stresses of daily life: a misplaced key, a person in the "8 items or less" checkout lane with 12 items in the cart, a neighborhood dog walking on their lawn.

Believe it or not, there's an explanation for these outbursts. Small, insignificant situations are the very ones the patient would have handled without a thought in the past. But now, every one of these actions, every one of these situations may uncover his inability to deal with simple stress and frustration.

Another point: How you react to these outbursts will greatly influence the head-injured person's behavior. Do your best to stay calm and speak in a soothing voice; redirect the person quickly by changing the topic and finding a quiet, distraction-free environment. It's important to reward and reinforce appropriate behavior, but not punish for verbal outbursts. For example, a decrease in verbal outburst might be rewarded with increased television time or a movie, while continued outbursts are met with no reward. Reinforce the positive!

2. "Breaking Down the House" or Physical Outbursts

Throwing an ashtray, breaking a vase, or hurling spaghetti against the wall can be triggered by events that normally would not cause such behavior. Head injured survivors have difficulty controlling their impulses. Noisy, chaotic and frustrating circumstances tend to increase the chance that such an outburst may occur. These outbursts are not premeditated but are more like an "automatic reflex".

3. "I'm Most Important" or Egocentricity

Your head-injured loved one has indeed gone through a terrible experience, and he needs to talk about himself, about the pain he's been through, to release some of that tension. But his egocentricity can also be a product of paranoia, of an inability to make a connection between logic and reality. Think of it. What if you lacked the ability to understand what someone was saying? What if you couldn't use your logic to realize that someone *really* isn't talking about you—or isn't trying to "get you"? All your focus would be on yourself. You would demand the attention of others. You would be completely unaware of other people's problems. And you would be functionally unable to share anything with anyone.

But egocentricity can hurt. One study found that a head-injured survivor's social network usually disintegrates after about six months—just enough time for friends to have new experiences that don't involve their head-injured pal, just enough time for them to see that their friend has become an angry, depressed individual who only wants to talk about himself and who doesn't care about them at all.

4. "Everything You've Always Wanted to Know About..." or Sexual Problems

Freud always claimed it was always on people's minds. But whether or not the idea of sex is a constant companion in everyday life, the libido is most definitely a factor in head injury. Sex drive may either increase or decrease. Some men's testosterone levels drop. Some women stop menstruating. These symptoms can have their roots in neurological damage to the hypothalamus (the regulator of sexual drive) or in purely psychological reactions. But cause isn't as important as result. The fact is that 50 percent or more of head-injured adults experience some form of sexual disturbance that sabotages their attempts to re-enter the real world.

Most head injuries occur to young men under 25—in

other words, to adolescents who are still developing, physically, mentally, *and* sexually. They are in a state of confusion; their hormones are surging. Add to this energetic libido the fact that many of these same head-injured teens come from unstable, unsupportive homes, and you have all the necessary ingredients for sexual dysfunction.

Many medications are given to head-injured survivors to prevent seizures, control blood pressure, or improve behavior. But they may also decrease feelings of sexuality or even cause impotence.

Role reversal also dampens sexuality between partners. What if your husband, who was always the one to handle the family's crises, large and small, became dependent after a head injury? You, the wife, may discover that being a 24-hour caregiver takes much of the thrill out of sex. Or what if it was your wife who was injured, and this formerly independent, accomplished woman now whines louder than your kids? These family dynamics need to be addressed before frustration, anger, and bitterness displace tenderness and love. Rehabilitation hospitals can help; so can family therapists. Don't be afraid to ask for help. The problem is much more common than you might think.

Compounding sexual dysfunction are the cognitive deficits that prevent a head-injured man or woman from correctly interpreting cues—sexual or otherwise. Picture this scenario: A head-injured man needing a bath and a shampoo goes to a singles' bar looking for a date. In his mind, he looks really terrific; he can't understand why the women are ignoring him. Instead of feeling good about his night on the town, he becomes anxious, frustrated and depressed.

Here's another scenario: A young head-injured woman believes the line a handsome young man gives her. She's in love; he tells her he loves her, too. But he dumps her after a one-night stand—and she can't understand why. She begins to hate herself; she gets depressed and withdrawn. It had to be something she did wrong....

On a different note, here's a story that connects sexuality with memory. It's an excerpt from "Issues of Sexuality in Head-Injured Adults," by Sheldon Berrol, M.D., as reprinted by the National Head Injury Foundation:*

---

*Reprinted by the NHIF with permission from *Sexuality and Physical Disability*, edited by David G. Bullard and Susan E. Knight, St. Louis: The C. V. Mosby Co., 1981.

HEADLINERS

ONE GIRL'S STORY

Jeanette never liked herself much; her self-esteem had never been high. But as she grew up, she discovered that by doing things for others, from donating to charity to being a thoughtful friend, she could actually find herself likeable. But after her head injury, Jeanette couldn't do the things that made her feel good about herself. Consequently, her self-esteem plummeted. She felt worthless. All the negative feelings that had been under wraps before the accident came out in full bloom. She became extremely depressed....

"Another patient of mine was constantly badgering his wife to engage in sex six, eight, and ten times a day. Every time she tried to do the wash he wanted sex, and she had a room full of unwashed laundry. In fact, his problem was one of memory. He had a very severe short-term memory problem in addition to retention memory deficits. He knew that he wanted to have sex but could not remember that he had had it...."

5. "I'm Right and There's No Use Arguing" or Rigidity and Inflexibility

As with most behavioral problems, rigidity and inflexibility have cognitive roots. Difficulty with problem solving, reasoning and memory often result in rigid and inflexible thinking and behavior. A head-injured person might be incapable of switching from one topic of conversation to another. His memory could be so poor that he is completely unaware that he's mentioned the same subject four times in the last five minutes. He might obsessively talk about a particular idea or concept for weeks at a time. Without the ability to think of multiple solutions to a single problem, the patient is "stuck" with a single, inflexible course to follow.

6. "Look Before You Leap" or Impulsive Behavior

"Think before you act" has no meaning to a head-injured person with an impulse-control problem. When the inhibiting neurotransmitters get damaged, a person's "social censor" —the ability to control oneself—flies out the window. Impulsivity mushrooms with stress, especially when the patient has to make a decision about something. She might "fly off the handle" at her husband when he asks her if she wants dinner now... She might type an entire five-page report, only to discover that she's misspelled a word on page two. Rather than salvage what she's done, she rips up the whole report and starts from scratch... She might decide to go up to the apartment of a man she just met on the bus, even though she knows nothing about him. It just seems like a good idea.

But there's still one aspect to behavior we have yet to explore. It's the single most important trait a head-injured person can have—but it's also one of the hardest to achieve....

"Who Am I?" or Developing Self-Awareness

FAMILY MEMBER: He just isn't the same person he was before.

INJURED PERSON: I don't know what she's talking about. I'm still me.

FAMILY MEMBER: He acts so crazy at times.

INJURED PERSON: I'm not crazy—she is.

Two different points of view—and each person feels he is right. But, unfortunately, there is no right—or wrong. It all comes down to perception. The family member is frustrated that the person she once loved has not only changed—he isn't even aware of it. Her head-injured spouse, however, is acting quite normal for someone in his condition. For him, self-awareness doesn't come easy—or fast. Not only is denial at work, but cognitive deficits as well. Listen to this sobering report:

A study of head-injured patients and their families *seven years* after the initial trauma found that the families felt their head-injured member was immature, childish—and unwilling to admit to any deficits.

But self-awareness is possible, as this woman's personal account from a National Head Injury Foundation article shows:

"For me, as for most people who have sustained a head injury, knowing what *was* made it difficult to accept what *is*. I had to learn to find a way to change that which should not be accepted, but also to compromise and accept that which could not be changed."

This woman learned self-awareness—and she is only one of thousands who have also succeeded in their quest. But they couldn't learn self-awareness on their own. They needed the help of a good rehabilitation program.

HARD, AIN'T IT HARD

Rehabilitation is probably the hardest thing that your loved one will ever do. It's harder work than preparing a paper for a conference. It's harder work than taking care of three kids. It's harder work than lifting weights and toting barges. It involves physical, emotional, and mental therapy. But, as the expression goes, you don't get something for nothing. Rehabilitation can be extremely rewarding for everyone—you, your loved one, and even society at large.

The good news is that rehabilitation programs today take behavioral and emotional problems into account. We'll discuss some of the newest techniques in Chapter Ten.

You now know how head injuries are caused. You know what happens when a head injury occurs. And you understand the symptoms that go beyond a "simple" bump on the head.

It's time now to talk about recovery, to find the reality behind your hope. It's time to journey toward getting well....

EIGHT

HOW TO PICK THE RIGHT REHABILITATION HOSPITAL

"Defeat is worse than death because you have to live with defeat."
—Bill Musselman, from *1,911 Best Things Anybody Ever Said*

- *MYTH:* One rehabilitation hospital is as good as the next.
- *MYTH:* If you don't have any money, forget about rehabilitation for a loved one.
- *MYTH:* Rehabilitation is just another way to take money away from families. My husband's just trying to get attention—like he always does.
- *MYTH:* My husband and I can take care of our head-injured child just fine at home, thank you.
- *MYTH:* My wife is severely head-injured. There's no hope for her. We might as well just give up.

If someone you love has had a head injury, chances are you've heard some of these comments—or you might even have said them yourself. It's understandable. With approximately 500 rehabilitation programs in the United States alone (plus three government-funded research and training centers), there's a dizzying array of rehabilitation hospitals to choose from—yet the family stress level may be so high that making the right decision seems an impossibility.

The fact is that good rehabilitation hospitals have been proven to really help. In a world where 80 percent of people

75

with head injuries recover their physical functions within a year but have lingering cognitive, behavioral, emotional, and social problems, good rehabilitation programs are needed more than ever. Above all, you need to know how to choose a rehabilitation hospital that meets your specifications.

THE FIFTEEN STEPS

All of us hope to function at our fullest potential—and head-injured survivors are no exception to that rule. They deserve a comprehensive rehabilitation program. The elements of that program may be as individual as the person himself, but we believe there are fifteen major components that every good rehabilitation program should include:

1. Evaluation and assessment of a patient's needs.
2. Physical independence activities dealing with mobility, strength, and endurance.
3. Activities of daily living such as dressing, grooming, personal hygiene, and feeding.
4. Cognitive rehabilitation to compensate for deficits in attention, memory, judgment, initiation, and planning.
5. Treatment for swallowing disorders.
6. Speech and language therapy for communication disorders.
7. Behavioral management and modification.
8. Sexuality counseling and support.
9. Social skills groups.
10. Family counseling to deal with adjustment to a loved one's disability.
11. Therapeutic recreation for teaching leisure skills.
12. Vocational assessment and retraining.
13. Re-entry into the community.
14. Patient and family education.
15. Alumni and support groups.

To further separate the myths from the realities of rehabilitation, here are a few more things to look for in a good program:

Reprinted from our article, "Head Injury: A Primer" in *Progress Report* magazine.

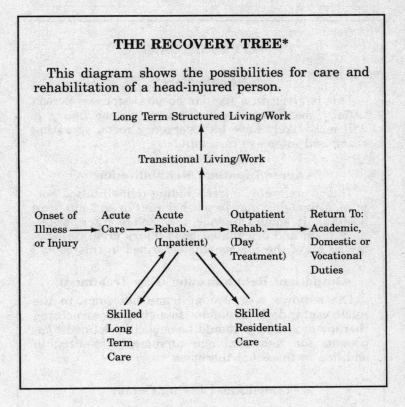

THE RECOVERY TREE*

This diagram shows the possibilities for care and rehabilitation of a head-injured person.

Long Term Structured Living/Work

Transitional Living/Work

Onset of Illness or Injury → Acute Care → Acute Rehab. (Inpatient) → Outpatient Rehab. (Day Treatment) → Return To: Academic, Domestic or Vocational Duties

Skilled Long Term Care

Skilled Residential Care

HOME, UNCOMFORTABLE HOME

The best intentions don't always yield the best results. As much as you'd like to take care of your loved one in the privacy of your home, it's a lot tougher than you think. Would you know how to get your husband into the shower? Could you change his clothes when he soiled them? How would you handle his excessive talking or a violent outburst?

Like it or not, you should know that home is not always the best place to be after a head injury. First of all, a hospital setting can supply the medical attention your loved one may need: An acute-care unit will stop infection from spreading, and reduce the brain swelling and pressure

Adapted from Interdisciplinary Teams and Medical Rehabilitation, Vangilder, C., and Fogt, M.

TYPES OF CARE

Acute Care

This is given in a regular hospital where a person usually goes immediately following a head injury. It will most likely have an emergency room, operating room, and intensive care unit.

Acute Inpatient Rehabilitation

This is preferably a freestanding rehabilitation hospital, although it may be a rehab unit in an acute-care hospital. It should provide a complete interdisciplinary team and designated head-injury program, supplying all of the components described in this book.

Outpatient Rehabilitation (Day Treatment)

The survivor will live at home but come to the rehab center daily for a four- to eight-hour structured therapy program. It should have clearly defined components for vocational and community re-entry, in addition to the usual therapies.

Transitional Living Center

This may be a house, group of apartments, campus setting, or ranch. The survivor lives in a structured environment where the necessary therapies can be provided. The goal is greater independence, but supervision, safety and support are very much at hand. The head-injured survivor might attend school or have a job.

Skilled Long-Term Care

Lower-level patients who cannot be cared for at home may require placement in a skilled nursing facility or nursing home. Many facilities have therapists on staff or who visit the facility daily.

buildup that can cause even more damage than the original injury.

Secondly, a rehabilitation hospital employs a staff that is specifically trained in head injury rehabilitation. They can supply the testing, the diagnoses, and the treatment program that you just don't have at home. They will also provide the facilities and structure—from physical therapy equipment to group social skills therapy—that your loved one needs for support, retraining, and, most importantly, successful re-entry into the community.

Above all, a good rehabilitation hospital will help train you so that when your loved one is returned home, you will be better able to cope with any aberrant behavior, functional problems—and stress that you may be feeling yourself. Knowing how to take care of a head-injured survivor will also help continue his rehabilitation, which doesn't stop when he does come home.

REFERENCES UPON REQUEST

Never underestimate the value of a recommendation. If your family doctor, a man or woman you trust, suggests a rehabilitation hospital, check it out. Other ways to get recommendations are:

1. Through your health or disability insurance company
2. Through your firm's human resources department
3. Through social workers in your area
4. Through other families within your community who have gone through the same experience as you
5. By contacting the National Head Injury Foundation at 333 Turnpike Road, Southborough, MA 01772 (508) 565-9950 or 1-800-444-NHIF.

BEST OUT OF THREE

Not all programs are the same. In the same way you'd seek a second opinion if you needed an operation, so should you research at least *three* rehabilitation hospitals. Although location is a factor, it shouldn't be the deciding one. It may be well worth the effort to travel that extra 100 miles or so for a program that offers exceptional service.

Try to get the names of some other families who have gone through the program at a particular hospital. Call or

HEADLINERS

SILENT EPIDEMIC

Why do you walk
The way that you do?
And why do you talk
But words are so few?
I don't understand your behaviors

Why can't you call
And just dial the phone?
In fact, I'm appalled
You can't live alone.
I don't understand your behaviors

Why do you toil
When baking a cake?
Can't measure the foil?!
You're so hard to take!
I don't understand your behaviors

Just stop acting crazy
Straighten up now
Perhaps you've turned lazy?
But sweat's on your brow
I don't understand your behaviors

Angry at me?
What did I do?
Oh, I failed to see
Beyond bodily clues
Teach me...to perceive your
behaviors
—A poem by Janice Cortis Kasowski, as reprinted in
The National Head Injury Foundation's "First Person
Accounts"

write them. See if their needs were similar to yours. Ask them what they were looking for in a program when their loved one was injured—and if they are pleased with the rehabilitation hospital they chose. Another telling point: Ask them if they would do anything differently if they could start over again.

ONE VISIT IS WORTH A THOUSAND WORDS

Let's face it: A rehabilitation hospital's brochure is going to put its best foot forward. How many of us have seen a hotel's lush brochure, complete with palm trees, ocean-view balconies, and spacious rooms—only to arrive and discover the cramped, slightly seedy reality? Although rehabilitation hospitals are scrupulous and federally regulated, they too want you to use their services; they too will use marketing tools so you will see them in the best possible light.

But seeing is believing and we cannot stress this enough:

VISIT ANY PROSPECTIVE FACILITY

Use your eyes. Inspect the rooms, the offices, the therapy areas. Make sure that the hospital is clean, and that there is sufficient space for all the different types of therapy that must be done to meet rehabilitation goals. Watch the staff. Are they attentive to their patients? Do they know where each patient should be at all times? Do the patients themselves have a schedule that they can follow, that, despite their deficits, has been taught to them in some form?

DOCTOR, DOCTOR

Yes, it's sad but true. Marcus Welby was the figment of a scriptwriter's imagination. But as busy, authoritative, and responsible as today's doctors are, they do not have to be the Invisible Man or Woman. Also, meet the doctor in charge of the facilities. If you were investigating RIOSA, you would make an appoint to meet with me, Richard Senelick. As Medical Director, I make it a policy to meet all interested families—and I answer any of their questions to the best of my ability. I know that if I were in their shoes, I'd want the same respect.

Not just the doctor, but also the staff may be interviewed and questioned. Don't be afraid to ask them

HEADLINERS

REHABILITATION CHECKLIST*

Some questions to help you in your rehab search:

- Will the family receive written reports on the patient's progress?
- How many individuals with head injury has the hospital treated since they started the program?
- What is the average length of stay? Who determines it?
- Are previous medical records incorporated into evaluations and treatment?
- What is the weekend/weeknight program?
- If the family is at a distance, what is the protocol for telephone contact?
- How often is a comprehensive re-evaluation done?
- What is the hospital's philosophy on medication?
- Can the hospital meet the family member's specific and individual needs, including tracheostomy, feeding tube, bowel and bladder control, loss of vision, shunt, and more?
- Is there post-discharge followup?
- If a legal settlement is obtained during a person's stay in the program, will the program expect higher reimbursement than that quoted upon admission?

about their credentials and experience. How accessible are they? Do they seem sensitive to your needs? Do they treat their patients with compassion? Does the hospital use a team approach, in which cognitive retraining, behavioral therapies, social skills training, vocational and physical therapies are all equally stressed with everyone working together.

Another telling point: Check to see if the rehabilitation hospital is licensed via CARF (Commission on Accreditation of Rehabilitation Facilities). In the same way that some doctors are board-certified, rehabilitation hospitals can also have that "extra edge" of expertise.

*Printed in The National Head Injury Foundation's "What to Look for When Selecting a Rehabilitation Facility: A Working Guide."

MONEY WON'T BUY EVERYTHING, IT'S TRUE

Finances are always the bottom line. But bottom lines can be explored, analyzed, and understood. The rehabilitation hospitals you are checking out should have case workers who will be individually handling your situation, guiding you through the maze of legal and insurance matters. They will keep you informed about progress, financial resources, insurance payments, and the exact cost of the program over and above what is paid by insurance. In their article "Advocating for Funds," The National Head Injury Foundation suggests that financial assistance can also be obtained from such public programs as Supplemental Security Income (SSI), the Social Services Block Grant, Veteran's Benefits, and Vocational Rehabilitation. Private sources include Workers Compensation, Auto No-Fault and Liability, Accident and Health Insurance, Preferred Provider Organizations, Health Maintenance Organizations, Short- and Long-Term Disability, Reinsurance and Self-Insurance, as well as funds from private philanthropic organizations.

DRUG DEALING

It's sad, but true. As we have seen throughout this book, drug and alcohol abuse go hand-in-hand with head injury. Make sure that your rehabilitation hospital of choice has access to support groups to help patients deal with substance abuse—and that it offers patients more positive ways to cope, including relaxation strategies and the solid support of peers. Further, the rehabilitation program should also incorporate a behavior and environment management program, in which drugs are locked up to keep the patients' surroundings safe.

A FAMILY AFFAIR

Illness is never a solitary pursuit. Whether it's a broken leg, major depression, or a head injury, the patient's family (or a significant other) will always be involved. Make sure that the rehabilitation hospital includes you in the treatment team, explaining procedures, medical terminology, and prognosis for recovery. Find out if family therapy or meetings are routinely scheduled, and if the staff teaches you as well as the patient. After all, you will ultimately be the responsible caregiver.

INSTINCTIVE BEHAVIOR

When it comes to childrearing, Dr. Spock, has said, "Trust your instincts." The same goes for your head-injured loved one—and the rehabilitation facility you ultimately choose. Trust your feelings. Observe how welcome the place makes you feel...how professional the staff appears...how clean, safe, and efficient the surroundings are...how the staff treats you, your loved one, and other patients. It's true that you will need education in caring for a head-injured loved one, but don't underestimate the power of love. It can go far.

But there's more. In order to fully understand a rehabilitation facility, you need to know exactly who is on staff—and why. We'll review this next....

NINE

THE TREATMENT TEAM

"I don't think of her as my physical therapist. I think
of her as my friend."
          —A 36-year-old housewife and patient at RIOSA

• The physical therapist lifts his arm slowly and helps
  him maneuver from the wheelchair to the rocker for
  vestibular stimulation.
• The occupational therapist helps her become more aware,
  providing education and training in tasks of daily living
  including oral hygiene, grooming, and dressing.
• The speech therapist puts her hands on either side of
  her mouth, helping to promote normal oral muscle activity.

These are descriptions of rehabilitation in action. Physical therapists, occupational therapists, speech therapists
and others—all work together to provide the best possible
care and treatment for head-injured patients.

But, as you could tell when you read over these statements, rehabilitation can sound rather complex and unin-
viting. You already know how to pick a good facility. Now
it's time to actually enter the maze and discover the cast of
characters who work in concert to help your loved one as
best they can.

THE MEMBERS OF THE TEAM

The Captain: The Rehabilitation Physician

A neurologist specializes in disorders of the nervous
system, specifically the spinal cord and the brain. A physi-

HEADLINERS

SIX GOLDEN REHABILITATION RULES FOR PATIENT CARE

1. Every patient needs to be given a chance at good rehabilitation before concluding that no change is possible.
2. Rehabilitation is a long process.
3. Treatment should not focus predominantly on physical deficits.
4. Recreational and vocational rehabilitation are essential.
5. Rehabilitation must include and involve the patient's family.
6. You *must* treat the patient as if he is going to improve.

---

atrist is a doctor of physical medicine and rehabilitation. In addition to treating medical problems, these doctors might also oversee the rehabilitation hospital's physical, occupational, and speech therapists. Either or both doctors may direct the medical and rehabilitation care of the head-injured patient including the management of medications.

Pitcher: The Neuropsychologist

Neuropsychologists specialize in the relationship between the brain and behavior. They perform those numerous neuropsychological tests we discussed in Chapter Four, as well as evaluate a patient's cognitive abilities, his behavior, and any psychological problems he might have. This information will be passed along to the entire team—as well as to the patient and his family—to help determine a specific rehabilitation program.

They also conduct group and support therapies, as well as individual and family therapy. These therapies frequently involve the establishment of a behavior management program.

First Baseman: The Physical Therapist

His or her function is exactly as it sounds: to treat the head-injured person's physical deficits. This might mean teaching the patient to:

- Walk again
- Use a wheelchair on various terrains
- Get in and out of a wheelchair
- Maintain normal posture

A physical therapist also works on improving muscle tone, flexibility, balance, coordination, movement, energy endurance, and strength via various exercises and activities. He or she will work closely with the other "basemen."

Second Baseman: The Occupational Therapist

The picture most people see when they envision an occupational therapist at work is someone supervising a room full of hospital-robed patients making pottery vases and potholders. In reality, an occupational therapist is involved in every aspect of a head-injured patient's rehabilitation. Finger and hand agility. Perception. Cognitive functioning. Eye-hand coordination. Activities of daily living (ADL) functioning, relearning everything from how to take a bath to how to cut a steak. All these and more are the province of the occupational therapist. And, oh yes, in improving social interaction and thought-processes within groups, an occupational therapist just might have some pottery sessions.

Shortstop: The Speech Therapist

A speech therapist knows a lot more than how to correct a lisp. Her responsibilities include evaluating and treating deficits in the areas of speech production, language expression, comprehension, reading, writing, and even swallowing. She is also a key player in the rehabilitation of cognitive functioning, working on the patient's attention and memory skills as well as his skills in abstract reasoning and decision making. In addition, the speech therapist pays attention to social skills, helping the head-injured patient re-master the art of conversation. Finally, since behavior and cognition are so interrelated, the speech therapist often assists in developing and implementing the patient's behavior management program.

Third Baseman: The Rehabilitation Nurse

Nurses are key players in any hospital program, and a rehabilitation nurse has a particularly vital function. She tends to the patient's needs and comforts, but that's just the beginning. In addition, she helps evaluate and treat his physical health, his problems with personal hygiene, and his impaired bladder and bowel control. She passes along her information to the attending physicians and the other members of the team. She's involved in helping the patient reach his therapy goals during non-therapy hours. (For example, if the physical therapist is teaching the patient how to transfer himself into and out of his wheelchair, the nurse will help him practice his transfers in the evenings.) The nurse also plays an important role in social skills training, such as helping the patient relearn to eat, mingle socially, and function with others.

Outfielder: The Respiratory Therapist

Unless a patient is severely head-injured, this therapist may only be involved in the early stages of recovery. He or she will be on call if the patient has trouble breathing or coughing, or needs tracheostomy care. The expert care of a respiratory therapist frequently prevents infection and complications.

Outfielder: The Clinical Dietitian

Everyone has to eat right—including head-injured patients. A dietitian is especially important for them, because nutritional needs can change drastically after an accident. A person might have lost a great deal of weight in the early stages of recovery, especially if he or she was in a coma; they will need more food to help their physical recuperation. A dietitian will also detail a diet for those head-injured survivors who cannot control their eating, as well as special diets for those with bowel or swallowing problems.

Outfielder: The Vocational Specialist

Independence is the goal of any good rehabilitation program. In order for a head-injured person to achieve a sense of independence and self-esteem, he or she must learn to live in the outside world. That's where vocational specialists comes in. If the patient is a student, they will evaluate

HEADLINERS

REHABILITATION STAFFERS ARE PEOPLE, TOO

There's no doubt about it. Working with a head-injured patient can be frustrating. Inappropriate remarks, emotional mood swings, confusion, cognitive failings—all these can take their toll. As any family member knows, you need time out, too.

The staff must make a commitment not only to help a patient, but to help themselves as well. Social support systems. Staff social functions. Staff meetings to let off "steam." Plus further education to:

- Keep themselves stimulated
- Help the patients even more
- Remind themselves of why they wanted to enter the rehabilitation field in the first place: to help someone in need.

his academic performance, develop an individualized education "package" for him, and help place him in a school when the time comes.

If the patient is an adult, vocational specialists will help him or her with career goals. They will work with the speech therapist to build up attention and concentration skills, cooperativeness, the ability to follow directions, and more. They will teach specific job skills—from typing and hairdressing to sewing and welding—if the patient is unable to return to the job he or she held before the accident.

Outfielder: The Rehabilitation Counselor

Like the neuropsychologist, the rehabilitation counselor deals with the psychological and behavioral ramifications of a head-injured patient. But the rehab counselor is also involved in the patient's social behavior—and his history. These counselors interview both the patient and his family, asking detailed questions about the patient's personality before the trauma, his habits, his education, and his development. The rehab counselor's assessment analyzes the family structure as well as the family's goals for their loved one. This assessment helps the staff and family work together; it helps both of them with long-term hopes and goals.

Outfielder: The Recreational Therapist

Leisure time is as important as work, and leisure time can also be educational. Recreational therapists help patients re-enter their community. They initiate field trips to, say, supermarkets or restaurants. They organize group events, such as gardening, cooking, arts and crafts, or music appreciation. All of these activities provide opportunities for patients to practice new or relearned skills in functional, real-life situations. Recreational therapists also help patients use community resources, such as public transportation or the public library, to help make re-entry into the real world as smooth as possible.

Team Manager: The Case Manager

The glue that holds the pieces together. The mechanism that turns the wheel. The umbrella that deflects the rain. The case manager is all this and more. He or she is the liaison between the patient and his family, between the family and the rehabilitation staff, the family and their insurance companies—and always on an ongoing and dynamic basis. Case managers explain to families what their loved one's rehabilitation program hopes to accomplish. They help the family find financial resources to pay for rehabilitation. They help the family find support groups to deal with their own stress. They continue to assist the patient and his family over the long haul, helping the family cope with the patient's re-entry into the community. In short, whenever the family has a problem, a question, or a concern, their first stop is the case manager. Good rehabilitation hospitals have a case manager assigned to every patient.

Above all, there is you—the family. As the people closest to the head-injured patient, you are the most influential and important team members of all. You should be included in all major decisions and aspects of the rehabilitation program, not just for your own sake, but also for your head-injured loved one. Your feedback and information will help the health professionals do their job better.

HEADLINERS

AN EXAMPLE OF HOW A REHABILITATION NURSE CONTINUES THERAPY GOALS:

Activity:
Feeding
Considerations:
Insure that the patient is in an adequate **position** before **feeding** to facilitate good **swallowing**. Set up food for **visual** field work and one-sided neglect.
Activity:
Dressing
Considerations:
Insure room is set up so patient can **find** clothing easily. Have patient **pick out clothing and organize** what they will wear that day. Start clothing on affected side and assist patient to **use the unaffected arm** to pull clothing up. Help **sequence** through activity
Activity:
Grooming
Considerations:
This activity provides **tactile self-stimulation** and increases **body awareness** when the patient is assisted through the **task.**
Note: **Interdisciplinary goals are in boldface.**

A TEAM APPROACH

The baseball analogy might be stretching it, but the fact remains that every member of the team works together in an interdisciplinary approach. A baseball game isn't played by one person alone, nor can a successful rehabilitation program be carried out single-handedly.

For example, several therapists may address the patient's *sequencing skills* in different ways, with everyone working toward a common goal. The physical therapist helps him with the sequencing skills he needs in order to transfer himself from bed to wheelchair and wheelchair to bed. The occupational therapist helps him with the sequencing skills involved in preparing a meal. The speech therapist helps him in sequencing words and sentences to write a letter.

Another type of treatment is called co-treatment. This

involves two therapists working together with a patient, during a single treatment session, to achieve a common goal. Co-treatment can enhance the patient's level of functioning by simultaneously addressing many deficits that interfere with her ability to perform. For example, at meal time, if the patient has trouble staying awake and also has episodes of choking, then her co-treatment might involve both a physical therapist and a speech therapist. The physical therapist would help her to sit upright with proper balance and head control, which would raise her level of alertness and make her less likely to choke. Simultaneously, the speech therapist would coach her in safe, efficient swallowing techniques.

THERAPY BY ANY OTHER NAME

In addition to the team approach and co-treatment, there is also intensive one-on-one therapy. Physical and occupational therapists might work alone for a concentrated dose of coordination and muscle strength; they use a lot of mat work and stretching. The speech therapist works alone in a distraction-free environment to improve attention and decrease distractibility, or to focus on specific cognitive or communication skills with the patient.

STRENGTH IN NUMBERS

Groups can sometimes accomplish what individuals alone cannot. There is strength in numbers—plus peer pressure and understanding. Therefore, group therapy is another approach often used, to:

- Offer valuable support among others in the same situation.
- Help develop social skills.
- Create empathy and sympathy—two strong feelings that will help the patient re-enter the community.
- Facilitate awareness of deficits by observing and critiquing others with similar problems.

From the case manager to the dietitian, this is the rehabilitation team you and your loved one will get to know well. But there's still more. Before you can freely walk through the rehabilitation maze, you must understand the process. Read on. . . .

TEN

THE PROCESS OF REHABILITATION

"The sooner you get someone into the rehab setting, the more you can help them regain some level of independence."

—Mary Ann Harvey, R.N., Coordinator
of the High Observation Unit of RIOSA

You didn't think it could happen. You never gave it another thought. Head injuries occur to other people, other lives. But it did happen. You went camping with your family that vacation weekend. You couldn't sleep that first night. You crept out of your sleeping bag. You crawled out of the tent, carefully, silently, so you would not wake your family. You stared at the dying embers of the fire. You put on your hiking shoes and walked to the left, to the appealing stretch of trees and starlit night. You were looking for the Big Dipper when your foot slipped. You reached the end of the path; the edge of the cliff awaited. You fell, stunned and surprised, barely uttering a word, until you hit the bottom. Your head struck a rock....

Next you hear the sirens above the cliff. You see a whirring red light. But where are you? What are those lights? Who are you?...

You lose consciousness again. You are taken to the emergency ward of a nearby hospital. Your spouse sits next to your bed, holding your hand and crying. Your children are outside. But you are still unconscious. Unaware or not sure of where you are, who you are, and what happened to bring you to this place.

What happens to 500,000 people a year has also happened to you. You have had a head injury....

A diagnosis is made: a severe closed head injury, the result of falling down the cliff and striking your head. A large hematoma must be surgically removed from the left frontal lobe. Possible frontal, temporal, and diffuse damage. The prescription? Acute care for several weeks. Transfer to a rehabilitation hospital when condition is no longer acute. Probable deficits include short-term memory loss, paralysis of the right side, perception and comprehension problems, possible loss of executive functions, and disinhibition. Long-term outlook: guarded if patient awakens after surgery and shows steady improvement.

This is only a scenario, but it could happen. In fact, it did happen to one particular patient at RIOSA. His condition is currently stable, and his wife is in continual touch with his case manager. She now understands the program, the procedures, the chances of recovery. She is involved with every aspect of her husband's rehabilitation. She is a member of the interdisciplinary team.

Right now, you might have a case manager working with you at a particular rehabilitation hospital. You might understand exactly what is going on with your head-injured loved one. But if you are still confused by the terms medical professionals use, if you are overwhelmed by the day-to-day rehabilitation routines, if you cannot comprehend how each therapy works, then read on. We will be your case manager guides, showing you rehabilitation in action—and how the various therapies work toward a common goal: helping the head-injured patient achieve independence and live life to the fullest potential.

ACUTE DISTRESS

In an ideal world, rehabilitation starts in the emergency room as you are wheeled in, possibly unconscious or confused, after your accident. A neurologic team performs a wide range of diagnostic tests, including a blood workup, CT scans, MRIs, and sensory-motor exams; you will be classified according to the Glasgow Coma Scale, which helps determine the severity of your injury and the deficits you are most likely to encounter as you progress. The neurologic team also determines if there is any swelling, fluid buildup, and resulting intracranial pressure, as well as any of the other secondary physical symptoms we described in Chapter Five.

HEADLINERS

Sometimes emergence from a coma may be assisted by a tug at the emotional heartstrings—at least that's what John P. LaRue, M.S., discovered when he invented a storybook cassette player that a 2-year-old could control with a nudge. For one particular 2-year-old, the cassette played a bedtime story read by his parents. The child eventually understood the stimulus-response connection between nudging the cassette into action and hearing his parents read a story—a crucial first step as he came out of his coma.

At this point, rehabilitation consists of proper positioning and movement to prevent bed sores, weakened muscles, and spasticity. Sensory stimulation—either conversation, soft music, or touching—might be enacted. Vital signs are carefully watched. A respiratory therapist may help you breathe with a ventilator; she or he will help you cough to clear your lungs and avoid the risk of pneumonia.

At RIOSA we have what is called a "High Observation Unit." Patients can be brought in to this unit much earlier than in most rehabilitation hospitals. Here, the patient is dressed every day—shoes, shirt, socks—even if he can't lift his head or move his body. His hair is washed and groomed. Vital signs and life support systems are, of course, constantly monitored, but in addition, routines are established: speech, occupational, and physical therapy is begun. As Mary Ann Harvey, the R.N. Coordinator of this unit, told *Progress Report* magazine, "We begin our work with patients early in the process of recovery, before skills deteriorate even further."

Eventually, the patient's condition stabilizes. Surgery has been performed. His brain is healing; pressure is down. He is in a confused, agitated state and ripe for more complex rehabilitation. He is transferred from the "High Observation Unit" to a regular room, or from an intensive-care unit to a rehabilitation hospital.

REHAB AT WORK

We confess: We're not magicians. Nor are we miracle-workers, rainmakers, or alchemists who make gold out of

HEADLINERS

BRAIN PLASTICITY

"Plastic" is not just an environmental pollutant. It can actually be a good word—especially when it comes to the brain. Read on:

The brain is *not* a muscle. You can't exercise it to make it better. But we can teach compensatory strategies. We can take advantage of returning nerve cells. We can redirect messages to other pathways in the brain. This is especially successful in young children because of the plasticity of their brains.

Children, as a rule, are more flexible than adults. They are constantly discovering the world and they are delighted by surprises. Because they haven't completely developed, their brains are more flexible, too. Pathways can be better redirected. Some children who sustain serious head injury when they are small grow up to be completely normal adults—without any deficits at all.

stone. But we are experienced caregivers who like what we do. We are professionals, helping patients compensate for deficits and live to their fullest potential. We are educators, teaching families how to cope with a head-injured loved one. We are knowledgeable and responsible—and we can help a head-injured patient and his family more than any traditional hospital, emergency ward, or nursing home can.

With all our knowledge, research, and ability, we don't know exactly *why* rehabilitation works—we just know that it does. We can't measure in exact terms a lot of what happens with a head-injured patient. So much of the work we do is intangible; so much of the injury itself is intangible. In fact, during the first six months after an injury spontaneous recovery can occur. This natural healing might take place up to two years after the injury. There is no rhyme nor reason, no predictable day of the month when one patient gets his memory back, when another patient begins to understand what she reads, when a third patient stops seeing double.

No, we can't make spontaneous recovery happen. Nor can

we bring dead nerve cells back to life. But what we *can* do is:

1. *Evaluate a patient's needs and establish his goals.* In traditional medicine, taking down a medical history and performing a physical exam may be enough to determine a diagnosis and treatment plan. But, as you saw in Chapter Nine, rehabilitation uses the team approach—which can mean up to 12 different staff members, therapists, physicians, and psychologists, who will meet with the patient and his family and analyze his condition, a process that can take anywhere from five to ten days to complete. Once everyone has had a chance to discuss their evaluations, a plan is made—a well-informed and well-thought-out rehabilitation program that takes into account the patient's individual needs, potential, and future goals. This process is also dynamic. It is flexible and ready to be changed when the patient's condition changes.

2. *Prevent medical complications.* Even the comatose, severely head-injured patient can benefit from rehabilitation focusing on nutrition, skin care, bladder and bowel care, and prevention of muscle breakdown. Without proper care, a patient can deteriorate and never reach his full potential.

3. *Teach a patient compensatory strategies to make up for his disability.* No, we can't help nerves grow or fractures heal, but we can help the patient reach his maximum potential with a returning function. We can teach strategies to compensate for disabilities.

4. *Maximize those abilities that do start to come back.* It's true that many patients might not be able to use their legs again. They might remain paralyzed from the waist down. They might never be able to pronounce words coherently. They might never be able to keep organizational responsibilities straight. But if memory starts to come back, it can be used to help organize thoughts. If problem-solving skills start to return, they can be used to help the patient cope with getting around in a wheelchair. This kind of rehabilitation is, in the truest sense, a matter of accentuating the positive.

And we do see positive results. We know that we make an impact, because many patients do get better. Some get jobs. They can be independent at home with a minimum amount of supervision.

It makes sense. We keep patients safe in a structured, secure environment. We are consistent in our methods. We teach awareness. We repeat our lessons over and over again—as often as it takes. And, above all, we emphasize *function* above theory or psychology. Helping a head-injured patient, say, get to a bank, sign a check, and deposit it will do more for his self-confidence, self-esteem, and functional abilities than all the tests, mazes, fill-in-the-blanks, and therapeutic analyses in the world.

But along with consistency, function, repetition, and structure, there are methods to our "madness"—the actual techniques used in rehabilitation. Let's briefly review them now and see how they work.

MIND OVER MATTER, OR COGNITIVE REHABILITATION

Knowing isn't necessarily thinking. Cognitive rehabilitation isn't just involved with memory function, executive function, problem-solving skills and comprehension. It also deals with attention and concentration, appropriate behavior and social communication, activities of daily living and functioning in the real world—to the best of a head-injured person's ability. In fact, knowing is a broad term, involving *all* the disciplines of rehabilitation. As Drs. George Prigatano and Yehuda Ben-Yishay define it in "Cognitive Remediation," their article in *Rehabilitation of the Adult and Child Brain with Traumatic Brain Injury*, cognitive rehabilitation is "The amelioration of the deficits in problem-solving abilities in order to improve functional competence in everyday life situations."

Here's an example of cognitive rehabilitation in action:

After his accident, fifteen-year-old Charlie couldn't read. After extensive testing, our team agreed that his primary problem was paying attention. He couldn't stay focused on the task at hand.

In fact, Charlie's attention span was so limited that Beth, his speech therapist, could only work with him in five-minute increments. She might have booked 45 minutes a day for therapy, but half of those minutes would be "break time." She'd bring him back into focus by various cognitive remediation techniques, including:

• *Cueing.* If they were working with a workbook, and Charlie became distracted, Beth would cue him back to the appropriate point. Other cueing methods include wrist-watches with alarm systems set to go off in ten-minute increments and big, brightly colored signs stating, "Time to pay attention!"

• *Strategy teaching.* In the best of all possible rehabilitation worlds, the patient and the therapists work together to come up with strategies to cope with the patient's limitations. In Charlie's case, he and Beth listened to "Books on Tape" in five-minute intervals; they'd then read those same sections in a book. Every five minutes, Charlie's alarm clock would ring—reminding him to pay attention. And every half hour, he'd take a break. He and Beth would chat about the books he used to read, his war heroes, even the latest movies. After ten minutes, they'd go back to the task at hand, again setting Charlie's watch for five-minute intervals.

Eventually, Charlie's attention span grew. He no longer needed to be reminded every five minutes to stay focused. He no longer needed long breaks. His problem-solving skills got better, his memory improved, and he was able to read and understand large-print books. And, as an added plus, Charlie also improved his social skills—he was able to discuss books, movies, and life at large with anyone who asked.

• *Altering the environment.* Whenever Beth or anybody else worked with Charlie, they did so in quiet, distraction-free rooms with subdued lighting. The fewer distractions, the fewer stimuli that could tear Charlie's attention away.

• *Overlearning.* New information is "packaged" in what scientists call *engrams.* These engrams are stored in the brain, ready to be "opened" at a memory cue. But head-injured patients with memory problems need to create new engrams—or at least new pathways to "unlock" them from storage. Using repetition, patience, consistency, structure, and simple explanations, a therapist will teach something over and over again—until it has become an engram.

Reading one particular children's book out loud to Charlie over and over again made him finally remember it. When he read the book to himself, he continued to remember. Words began to make sense. What he "overlearned," he carried over to other books. His attention was getting better; his concentration was focused because he now understood what he was reading—and he enjoyed it.

HEADLINERS

TAKE ME FOR A RIDE IN YOUR CAR, CAR

Some memories are so deep, so ingrained, and so overused in the past, that brain damage will not destroy them. These "packets of information," or engrams (see "Overlearning," below) include singing the words to "Happy Birthday," a short prayer, a multiplication table—even driving a car.

It's not uncommon for many head-injured people to appear to be able to drive a car. Automatic and overlearned responses may suffice under "ideal" driving conditions. However, problems with reaction time, judgment and safety awareness can make "real life" driving highly dangerous.

• *Chain of events.* We don't even think about such automatic routines as, say, brushing our teeth or putting the water on to boil for coffee. But for someone with a cognitive deficit, each step must be spelled out—in sequence. Listen to the 12 steps needed simply to make a peanut butter and jelly sandwich to have with a glass of milk and some chips (taken from a RIOSA orientation booklet):

1. Must find peanut butter and jelly on shelf of refrigerator and move them to the counter.
2. Must get a knife out.
3. Must get a loaf of bread out of the pantry.
4. Must get a plate and glass out of the cupboard.
5. Must get milk out of the refrigerator.
6. Must get chips out of the pantry.
7. Must get a napkin out.
8. Must put peanut butter on bread.
9. Must put jelly on bread.
10. Must put two pieces of bread together.
11. Must put milk in the glass.
12. Must put peanut butter and jelly and milk back into refrigerator.
13. When finished eating must put dishes in the sink.

In addition to writing these steps down, a therapist will recite them out loud to cue the patient, acting as a "stage manager," watching the patient cope with each step. The therapist also has to make sure that counters and cabinets aren't cluttered, that food items have easy-to-read labeling, that the patient knows how to scan from left to right, top to bottom, to locate the items needed. It's no wonder that head-injured survivors can become frustrated and depressed! Simple chores and tasks have become elaborate productions....

Unfortunately, even if a head-injured survivor finally learns how to make a peanut butter and jelly sandwich or how to brush his teeth, chances are he'll forget some of what he learned when he gets back home. Why? Because the structure, quiet, and consistency of the rehabilitation hospital is gone. There are many more distractions—plus the added stress of trying to "make it" in the real world.

But a solution is on its way....

SAT SCORES

SAT stands for Skills Acquisition Training; the term was coined by Norman Namerow, a neurologist specializing in rehabilitation. It aptly described our functional approach to head injury rehabilitation.

SAT is a total program, involving every member of the team, all of them joined together to retrain a person to function in the real world. Rather than teach someone, say, problem-solving skills on a computer or sequencing with numbered cards, therapists get the patients out in the world, doing what they'll be doing when they re-enter the community. Riding a bus. Reading a map. Going to the supermarket. Answering the phone. Learning functional skills.

The first order of SAT business is to discover the patient's strengths and weaknesses. Does he know how to act in public? Does he shout out rude remarks? Does he get confused? The weak areas are worked on, and the patient's strengths are used to build up his confidence and self-esteem. And, all the while, cognitive functions are being tapped....

When Charlie went out into the community, he became aware of his cognitive limitations in a way he'd never been able to in the hospital. He didn't know how to read a map to get to the library. He couldn't order lunch from a menu. But he was able to discuss books with the librarian when he and his group finally made it to the building. Because he could see both his problems and the positive results of his therapy in real, concrete terms, Charlie became motivated to keep going. Thanks to this functional approach, Charlie continues to improve.

And speaking of motivation, there's another area of therapy that is as important as cognitive rehabilitation. In fact, therapists consider it number one....

I AM I, AND YOU ARE YOU, OR
SELF-AWARENESS TRAINING

It's a reality we're all familiar with: If we deny we have a problem, we never solve it. If we don't feel motivated, we never get out of bed. A head-injured survivor is no exception. She must get beyond her denial. She must be motivated to reach her full potential. She must discover for herself what must be changed and how it can be changed—if she is to function in the real world. Each therapy, from individual counseling to social skills training, from speech and language therapy to behavior management, is designed to help a patient reach this goal. Here's an example of self-awareness training in action:

A woman in her early thirties had sustained a severe head injury. She had major muscular problems in her right arm and leg. During her daily physical therapy hour, she tried to do what the therapist asked her to do—with little or no enthusiasm. But during one particular session, she had the "subjective experience of coming into a normal postural alignment, with equal weight bearing through both sides of the body and with pelvis tilted forward." This position made her relax and, "at this precise moment, there was a clear change in her facial expression, which gave the therapist the impression that she was suddenly experiencing and recognizing an old muscular 'feeling' that had not been present for a long time. This was an extremely joyful experience for her and seemed to motivate her for more physical therapy." In fact, two and a half years after this self-awareness awakening, she had made considerable progress.

One of the techniques we have used to teach self-awareness is what we call "the apartment." Combining two rooms, we

Adapted from "Emotion and Motivation in Recovery and Adaptation After Brain Damage" by George P. Prigatano, from *Psychiatric Medicine*, Volume 7, 1989.

have constructed a studio apartment. There is a sink, an oven, a refrigerator, and cabinets. A private bath. A bed, a television, and a table and chairs. When a patient tells us that he doesn't need to be in a rehab hospital, that there's nothing wrong with him, that if he could just go home everything would be fine. We say, "Well. Why don't we spend some time in the apartment? I will stay with you, but I want you to show me that you can do everything on your own. If you do well, we will send you home...."

But the patient never doesn't do well. He sees, firsthand, that he can't cook or shower or turn on the television. He can no longer deny his problem; he has seen his deficits in action. Although this self-awareness can lead to depression, it usually won't last long. Combined with his busy routine and the support and praise of our staff, his new "self-awareness" will eventually give him the "push" he needs to learn how to live in his brave, new world.

ACTIONS SPEAK LOUDER THAN WORDS, OR BEHAVIOR MANAGEMENT

Pretend we're your former employers—and you're a head-injured patient wanting your old job back. Well, sure, we'll tolerate it if you're slow. We'll even tolerate you if you're not that smart. But we won't put out the welcome mat if you're argumentative, nasty, bossy, and difficult to deal with.

In other words, the biggest roadblock to independent living in society is not the physical deficits involved in head injury. It's not even the cognitive problems. It's behavior with a capital B.

We weren't the first ones to notice this. One study followed 44 young head-injured adults for two years after their injury. Though they had problems with family life, leisure time, and employment, most of the patients were able to adapt to their new situations—with one exception: They had lost their old friends because their behavior had changed so much.

But there is hope. Rehabilitation is a learning process, and behavior, too, can be learned—and, even more important, relearned. A study of brain-injured patients of all ages, from adolescence to adulthood, by Dr. William Burke and his associates at the New Mexico Highwatch Rehabilitation Center, showed this dramatically. The one element each person in this study had in common was the fact that they had each been considered unmanageable by other rehabilitation centers. Six months after participating in a highly structured behavioral management program, 95 percent of the patients were able to re-enter the community—and two-thirds of them were able to return to work! On an even more promising note, 80 percent of these same people continued to live independent, responsible lives one year later.

Here are some examples of how behavioral management can work:

• *Correcting problem behavior.* Tim was a model patient. He always came to his therapy appointments on time; he always tried to stay well groomed. But he had one big problem: he would have outrageous outbursts, and would occasionally make some dangerous threats. Ignoring them made it worse. So did anger. Only when the rehabilitation nurse carefully and calmly redirected him did Tim stop his outbursts.

• *Using a reward system.* At RIOSA, we use poker chips as rewards. Here's how it works: When a patient acts in socially appropriate ways during an activity, she gets a certain number of chips which can be cashed in for rewards. A reward might be an extra hour of television at night, or a field trip. But when the patient has an aggressive outburst, she simply doesn't get any chips for that session—and consequently, no reward. We never punish and take away chips. We reward appropriate hehavior.

• *Implementing self-monitoring techniques.* It's exactly what it sounds like: Self-monitoring helps patients learn appropriate behavior by thinking before acting out. Billy used a daily log to keep tabs on his behavior. The log was divided into two columns: Appropriate Behavior and Inappropriate Behavior. Billy would put an "x" in the column that applied after each therapy session. He also received his chips when he had three or more x's in the Appropriate Behavior column.

• *Utilizing negotiation.* Joan's therapist told her that if she just sticks to wheelchair practice for ten minutes, she'll get an extra chip.

• *Participating in support groups.* "Nobody understands" ..."I feel all alone"..."I wish there was someone I could talk to..." There's power in numbers—especially when the ranks are made up of people in the same situation as you. They can offer true empathy, understanding—and hope. Guided by therapists, head-injured patients get a chance to communicate with others in this group format. For the first time, they get to express their thoughts and feelings to people who have been there. Communication skills, social skills training, language skills, self-awareness—all these are developed within the group format. Support groups can involve everything from substance abuse problems to surviving in the world.

Behavior management permeates every aspect of the rehabilitation program. It's a useful approach no matter what the therapy. A patient gets a chip for a job well done. An occupational therapist calmly corrects the behavior of a rude teen. A physical therapist negotiates—and gets—an extra fifteen minutes to work on her patient's gait.

The results permeate the entire therapy program. If a patient feels better about himself, more confident and calm, he'll be more motivated to practice his cognitive skills. If he's getting along with others, he is less likely to act selfishly or throw a childish tantrum in front of his new friends.

Cognitive skills and behavior. Feelings and thoughts. You now know the basic elements behind a good rehabilitation program. Let's take a few moments to look again at what the other therapies work to accomplish:

"SPEAK EASY": SPEECH AND LANGUAGE THERAPY

You will find the speech-language therapist doing more than what her title might imply. She also teaches eating and swallowing techniques, and focuses on cognitive and communication skills—for instance, teaching a patient with verbal expression problems to use gestures or writing to help communicate his thoughts and needs. She will construct a "memory book" to help him keep track of what has gone on during the day. The memory book might include snapshots of family members, pets, and hospital staff, and brief notes made by a therapist or by the patient himself after a specific activity. It may also include:

• a calendar to help him recall the day and date
• sequencing instructions for various activities

- large printed cues—to use a knife and fork, for instance, or, in Charlie's case, to pay more attention

Speech and language therapy also involves the patient's family. Learning to read a paragraph is one thing, but a relative might want her loved one to be able to read his prescription or write down phone messages. A good therapist will concentrate on these particular, practical skills. One patient at RIOSA had little use of her hands. She had memory deficits and permanent speech damage. But she and her speech therapist were able to work out a communication technique. The patient would point out letters on a chart, spelling out words she wanted to say. The first time she was told that there was a chance she could communicate in the world, the patient spelled out her first message: "Please help me."

LEARNING BY DOING, OR OCCUPATIONAL THERAPY

During her occupational therapy hour, you'll find your loved one working on her safety awareness, her perceptual problems, her executive functions. But, while all these skill trainings are going on, the underlying object is to help her perform functional tasks. She might not see her blouse the way you see it; she might try to put her head through a sleeve. She might try to comb her hair with a toothbrush. Through occupational therapy sessions, she will not only learn, say, how to button her blouse, but the sequencing order for getting dressed.

Occupational therapists work on other activities of daily living such as grooming, bathing, and hygiene. If there is arm or hand weakness or a lack of coordination, the therapist will work on upper extremity exercises, perhaps using a splint or brace to decrease spasticity or increase upper extremity function.

LIFE IN THE REAL WORLD

At RIOSA, on any given day, you might get a whiff of a class's homebaked chocolate chip cookies fresh from the oven. You might notice the freshly seeded vegetable and flower gardens outside. You might see a group of head-injured patients clutching paper bags filled with groceries,

---

HEADLINERS

MEMORY BOOK ENTRIES

(NOTE: these are actual entries written by therapists after a session. Patients with memory loss problems will read through them later.)

7:50 AM: Lucy, I came in and we got you dressed. I helped you with your breakfast. Dr. Senelick came in. You spoke with him and showed him your fingernails. You watched TV. You're doing great. We love you.—Peggy

8:30 AM: Now you are sitting up in your chair making short work of your breakfast. There is absolutely nothing wrong with your appetite!—Nell

1:00–1:30 PM: Speech with Judy. You invited me to your party. We talked about what we would do at your party. We played the "Imagining" Game. You did well and earned 2 chips.

---

coming from a visit to the supermarket. Or they could be bringing souvenirs from a field trip to the nearby Alamo. You might overhear a patient pretending to call a perspective boss on a "fake" phone—learning what to say and how to say it. You might walk past a room where people are discussing the opening of the Berlin Wall. You might see a group barbequeing burgers on an outside grill—or playing volleyball in an open field. As you can see, activities of daily living (ADLs) are not just "tasks." They can actually be fun! But these ADLs do have a serious objective: teaching independence.

Recreational therapy. Music and art therapy. Vocational therapy. Budgeting classes. Social skills training. All these are designed to make the head-injured patient's re-entry into the community as smooth and stress-free as possible.

LET'S GET PHYSICAL, OR PHYSICAL THERAPY

Physical therapy is as much a part of the treatment package as anything else. Cognitive, behavioral, and self-awareness training is taught as patients learn how to

HEADLINERS

A DAY IN THE LIFE

Charles S.: Moderate Head-Injured 15-year-old Patient

7:15–7:45	Breakfast with other patients and staff
7:45–8:30	Activities of Daily Living (ADL) training (encompassing Occupational Therapy)
8:30–9:00	Current Events group (encompassing Occupational Therapy and Speech Therapy)
9:00–9:30	Wheelchair Mobility Group (Physical Therapy)
9:30–10:30	Speech Therapy
10:30–11:00	Occupational Therapy
11:00–12:00	Physical Therapy
12:00–12:30	Lunch
12:30–1:00	Rest
1:00–1:30	Rehabilitation Counseling (Individual Therapy)
1:30–2:00	Occupational Therapy
2:00–3:00	Social Skills Training (Encompassing Speech)
3:00–3:30	Rest
3:30–5:00	Community Reorientation Outing (Recreational Therapy)
5:00–5:30	Nursing (Physical Therapy and ADL)
5:30–6:00	Dinner
6:00–7:30	Rest
7:30–8:00	Survivors Support Group

transfer themselves from a wheelchair to a bed, from a sitting position to standing.

Physical therapy sessions also concentrate on range-of-motion exercises. As a result of their injury, many patients suffer from spasticity, or a prolonged contraction of the muscles—caused by disinhibition similar to the one that triggers socially inappropriate behavior. The physical therapist teaches patients how to relax and loosen these tight muscles.

Specific exercises can strengthen weakened muscles and increase overall endurance. Illness and inactivity dramatically reduce a person's endurance, making it difficult to get through the day without frequent rest periods. Once strength is adequate, it's possible to progress to walking. Initially, a patient may walk only between parallel bars and require a good deal of help from the therapist. Over time, he will graduate to a walker or a cane with four legs (quad cane), and hopefully on to independent walking.

A SPOONFUL OF MEDICINE, OR PSYCHOPHARMACOLOGY

Remember this slogan:
The best medicine is frequently no medicine at all.

Drugs can cloud already foggy minds. They can slow down the thinking process. They can cause damaging side effects. But if a patient is severely depressed or suicidal, if he has seizures, if his attention deficits or agitation border on the dangerous, that's a different story. Medicine that works on the chemical imbalances in the brain is necessary. Very briefly, here's a rundown of the medications commonly used in head-injury rehabilitation:

• *Antipsychotics.* These drugs work on the neurotransmitter called dopamine, stopping it from stimulating a dopamine receptor in the next nerve cell. These drugs have been used for schizophrenia for years. In head-injured patients, they effectively stop agitation, hyperactivity, hallucinations, and hostility. Unfortunately, while these drugs stop inappropriate behavior, they also cause memory, learning, and cognitive problems. They also have side effects, including movement disorders. They should be used sparingly and for as short a time as possible. *Common brand names: Thorazine, Haldol, and Prolixin.*

• *Beta Blockers.* These drugs are most commonly used for high blood pressure, migraines, and heart problems. They get their name by effectively "blocking" the beta-adrenergic receptors in the forebrain that carry the messages for anxiety, nervousness, and sweating. Because they block debilitating emotions, they may be used by musicians, actors, and other performers before going onstage. In head injuries they are used to treat agitation, aggression, and violence. Side effects include dizziness, apathy, impotence, and nightmares. *Common brand names: Inderal and Corgard.*

• *Psychostimulants.* These are mainly used for hyperactive children. But because they work on inattention, distraction, disorganization, impulsivity, mood swings, and apathy, they're sometimes given to head-injured patients. Psychostimulants increase the levels of the brain chemical dopamine—an inhibitory neurotransmitter. Their side effects include insomnia, anorexia, headaches, and irritability. *Common brand names: Ritalin and Cylert.*

• *Lithium.* Believe it or not, this drug was first discovered in spas in Ancient Greece; it was recognized early on as a stabilizing force. Lithium is commonly used for treating manic-depressive illnesses. In head-injured patients, it's used to stop aggressive behavior and instability. But it must be closely monitored; too much lithium can become toxic. Side effects include diarrhea, tremors, and at toxic levels, confusion and disorientation. *Common brand names: Lithium Carbonate and Lithobid.*

• *Dopaminergic Agents.* These drugs also work on the dopamine receptors at the synapses of the brain; they are used primarily in comatose and low-level patients to shorten coma and improve functioning. Side effects include dizziness, nausea, and confusion. *Common brand names: Parlodel and Permax.*

• *Anticonvulsants.* If a head-injured person suffers from seizures, these drugs can control them. They may also stop episodic explosive behavior—but primarily in patients with abnormal brain wave tests. Side effects include problems in cognition and learning. *Common brand names: Dilantin, Tegretol, and Depakote.*

• *Tricyclic Antidepressants.* A severely depressed patient might be given one of the tricyclic antidepressants, which are named for their three-ring molecular structure. If the medication works, it alleviates depression four to six weeks after the first dose. It must be given gradually until an appropriate level has been reached—and it must gradually be tapered off. Side effects include confusion and fatigue. *Common brand names: Tofranil and Elavil.*

In this chapter we've examined the many different types of therapy that are important to a patient's recovery. There remains, however, one more important area to discuss: the role of the family.

ELEVEN

THE FAMILY CIRCLE

"He looks like my husband, but he's not...My husband's gone."

—A wife of a RIOSA patient

- Statistics show that between 40 and 50 percent of all marriages in which one of the spouses has been head-injured end in divorce—and many professionals in the field put the percentage much higher.
- A study of 200 families in which one member has been head-injured found that the caregivers felt isolated and trapped. They felt neither married or single—and their sexual and emotional needs were unfulfilled.
- A study of wives one year after their spouses were head-injured discovered that they found their husbands selfish, childish, demanding, and dependent.
- The children of head-injured parents also suffer. Studies found that they are often anxious, irritable, depressed, unruly—and doing poorly in school. Why? As Michael E. Howard, Ph.D., writes: "Children catch it from both ends: they are obviously ignored by the head-injured patient who is hospitalized, but they are also often ignored by the spouse who is so caught up in his or her own grief."
- Since most head injuries occur to men, it's mothers who truly must "mother"—sometimes an entire family circle at once.
- Research has found that when someone suffers long-lasting harm from a head injury his family's sense of burden increases over time. At six months, relatives felt that their head-injured loved one's most outstanding

problems were loss of affection, poor control of temper, social withdrawal, lack of energy, cruelty, meanness, and unreasonableness. At one year, these same relatives felt just as strongly about these same issues. As more time elapsed, the relatives' capacity for coping with and accepting these problems *decreased*. A different study discovered that five years after an injury, 74 percent of relatives still said their head-injured family member's personality problems were tough to take.

Harsh statistics, but true. It is indeed, as Dr. Robert Sbordone states, it is the families who "are the real victims of a head injury." They too need attention and structure. They too need to be educated and trained. They too need nurturing and support. In fact, a good rehabilitation program spends extensive time working with the patients' families.

FAMILY TIES

One of the crucial elements for a good outcome is family support. In fact, Michael E. Howard, Ph.D., found that a key family member, one who is involved in all facets of the treatment plan, offering support, guidance, and help to his head-injured relative, is the single most important factor for successful rehabilitation.

But whatever your role in the new family dynamics, the best support you can give is educated support. And, in order to be educated and most helpful, you should expect your rehabilitation team to:

- Give *permission* to your family to ask questions—as many as you want, without feeling intimidated.
- Provide information and *more* information about head injury. The more you know, the better equipped you'll be to handle any problem that comes up.
- Find that key person in the family who will be a pillar of strength, support, and involvement—but, at the same time, find ways that he or she can get "time off."
- Assign one person, either a social worker or a case manager, to handle your family's questions or problems— from insurance and financial structures to family therapy referrals to help you all cope.
- Encourage support groups. Nothing will help a stressed-out and confused family more than a group of sympa-

HEADLINERS

LIKE A NOVEL

Ernest Hemingway suffered from a diagnosed depressive disorder—and alcoholism. Less well known was the fact that he had at least *five* head injuries during his life—one of them the result of a severe airplane crash in Africa. His increasing difficulty in writing, his excessive drinking, his depression, and even his ultimate suicide were possibly rooted in his head injuries. If only we knew then what we know now about head injury.

thetic, understanding peers who have "been there" themselves.
• Involve your entire family in all aspects of rehabilitation—from the confusion and isolation of intensive care through proper help in the activities of daily living.

FAMILY CRIES

A study of over 100 mothers of head-injured children by Ellen Zinner, Ph.D., et al, published in the National Head Injury Foundation's Newsletter, found that the biggest stressors for them were their child's behavior problems. One mother's complaint was "my son's temper—he gets loud and profane." Another mother complained of "mood swings in our daughter."

The second biggest stressors were family difficulties—the vicissitudes of life that continue even while tragedy strikes: a death in the family, poor sibling adjustment, financial burdens.

Other mothers worried about their child's recovery and the future. One mother feared, "the kind of life my son would have if I died, got sick, or emotionally burned out." Slow progress, the very real worry of rehabilitation expenses—all take their toll.

Most of these mothers felt that the most stressful time was right after the accident, while they were waiting to see if their child would live or come out of a coma.

However, there were a significant number of mothers

who felt just the opposite. For them, the most nerve-wracking time was after their child returned home: "the inability to go out since my son is at home and cannot be left unattended... the ongoing 'wear and tear' of living with a disabled person."

Others mentioned lack of communication between themselves and their child's doctors, and difficulty in finding others who understand what head injury is all about....

Finally, there was always that sadness—over what their child had lost—and over the lack of support from one-time friends and from other family members. As one mother wrote: "I have been bereaved. I have had time to realize that I no longer have the son I used to have, but one similar. I have begun to adjust after a period of depression."

You, too, can come out of the trauma intact. Here's some guidance to provide reassurance—and help make your adjustment easier and quicker. Adapted from "Living with the Characterologically Altered Brain Injured Patient" by Muriel D. Lezak, Ph.D., the six statements "family members need to hear" are:

1. Anger, frustration and sorrow are natural emotions for close relatives of brain-injured patients. Yes, it's true. You can grieve. You can feel angry at this person who changed your life. You can feel down in the dumps and even show a sour face to your head-injured loved one. Family caregivers who feel guilty when they feel angry, who chastise themselves for not being "perfect," will only get depressed, overwhelmed, and sick. After months of taking care of someone who is greedy, angry, childish, and unhappy, it makes absolute sense for you to occasionally say, "Be quiet!"

2. Caregivers must take care of themselves first. Look at any family rehabilitation booklet. Talk to any case manager or doctor. Before you can give to someone else, you must give to yourself. You must schedule free time. You must have "space." Some of the ways you can be good to yourself are:

- Eat right
- Express your feelings
- Seek professional help for emotional or adjustment problems
- Avoid drug and alcohol abuse
- Be kind to yourself

HEADLINERS

THE FIRST COPING STRATEGY—AND POSSIBLY THE BEST

Odysseus was a traveler—as Homer chronicled in his ancient classic, the *Odyssey*. He constantly ran up against disasters and villainous monsters—but always overcame the odds. Odysseus thought up one of his cleverest ruses as his ship was nearing Circe, the bewitching siren of the rocks. If he or his sailors heard Circe's song, they would become hypnotized and crash against the rocks in a horrible death. Rather than pray to the gods or tell his sailors to use self-control, Odysseus simply filled their ears with beeswax, effectively stopping them from hearing the siren's call.

The moral? Don't always try to make your head-injured loved one use self-control. Sometimes it's just a superhuman task. Instead, figure out a way to *circumvent* the problem.

- Buy yourself a present
- Exercise regularly to relieve stress
- Let others help
- Join a family support group
- Ask questions!!!

3. Trust your instincts. There will come a time when you must rely on your own conscience and judgment—even if it puts you in conflict with your loved one. Like the child who won't eat his vegetables, your brain-injured loved one might not know what's best for him. Combine his arguments with the well-meaning but contradictory advice other family members inevitably give, and you could remain frozen, unable to do anything, forever. Take charge. Armed with what you've learned, you can handle it.

4. The role changes that inevitably take place are emotionally draining—for everyone. You don't have to pretend that your spouse, the one-time wage-earner, responsible partner, and emotional helpmate, makes you happy—now that he has turned into a willful, dependent person. Nor do you have to "put on a happy face" when your adult, formerly independent child comes home bedridden and helpless. It's a terrible state of affairs. Roles that have been in place for years, family behaviors that were ingrained for so long they were automatic, family interactions that were once comfortably predictable, are no more. And because these changes occurred so suddenly, there's been no chance to adjust, no time for insights, no thoughts or game plan to help you carry on. Now, more than ever, you need to ask those questions—and seek the professional help of your case worker or hospital social worker.

5. *There may be little you can do to change your loved one—so there's no need to feel guilty when you see no improvement.* It's true. And, as hard-boiled as this statement is, it's also liberating. It frees you from the shackles of guilt. You can take care of yourself and rejoin the human race.

6. *When the welfare of your children is at stake, you must explore your divided loyalties and accurately weigh your responsibilities.* This is a painful issue—one that both families and case workers tend to gloss over. But the fact remains that if a brain-injured spouse has become abusive— even though it's through no fault of his or her own—you might have to figure out other living and caregiving arrangements.

FAMILY BINDS

Dr. Muriel Lezak, who came up with the above six statements families need to hear, has also outlined the six stages families typically go through when a loved one is injured. Here they are, as adapted by Dr. Michael E. Howard:

STAGE I

TIME SINCE HOSPITALIZATION: 1 to 3 months
FAMILY'S PERCEPTION OF PATIENT: A little difficult because of fatigue, inactivity, weakness, etc.
FAMILY EXPECTATION: Full recovery by one year
FAMILY REACTION: Happy

STAGE II

TIME SINCE HOSPITALIZATION: 1–3 months to 6–9 months
FAMILY'S PERCEPTION OF PATIENT: Not cooperating, not motivated, self-centered
FAMILY EXPECTATION: Full recovery—if he'll try harder
FAMILY REACTION: Bewildered, anxious

STAGE III

TIME SINCE HOSPITALIZATION: 6–9 months to 9–24 months; can continue indefinitely
FAMILY'S PERCEPTION OF PATIENT: Irresponsible, self-centered, irritable, lazy
FAMILY EXPECTATION: Independence—if they only knew how to help him
FAMILY REACTION: Discouraged, guilty, depressed, "going crazy"

STAGE IV

TIME SINCE HOSPITALIZATION: 9 months or later; can continue indefinitely
FAMILY'S PERCEPTION OF PATIENT: A different, difficult, childlike person
FAMILY EXPECTATION: Little or no change
FAMILY REACTION: Depressed, despairing, "trapped"

STAGE V

TIME SINCE HOSPITALIZATION: 15 months or later; usually time-limited
FAMILY'S PERCEPTION OF PATIENT: A difficult childlike dependent
FAMILY EXPECTATION: Little or no change
FAMILY REACTION: Mourning

STAGE VI

TIME SINCE HOSPITALIZATION: 18 to 24 months or later

FAMILY'S PERCEPTION OF PATIENT: A difficult child-like dependent
FAMILY EXPECTATION: Little or no change
FAMILY REACTION: Reorganization, emotionally, if not physically, disengaged

Typical, yes. But by no means absolute. Every family is unique—and the way you care for your head-injured loved one will reflect that individuality. Just as researchers have been able to generalize about the reactions a typical family might face, they've also been able to describe some typical behavior that helps create these negative reactions. Let's go over a few of these "brain teasers" now—with some "winning plays" to help you cope:

Brainteaser # 1: Overeating

Oh, the joys of food. There's nothing like a simmering soup on a winter's day, a refreshing iced drink when it's hot, a fresh baked cake... Unfortunately, these simple eating pleasures are much more complicated when it comes to head-injured patients. Initially, they *need* to eat, to make up for the nourishment they lost when first injured. Later, many caregivers are pleased to see that their patient is eating—especially when he might have spent months being fed in the hospital through a tube. A good appetite is a sign of health. And love, after all, is equated with food.

But this "health" can easily turn into an insatiable appetite—and your patient can get bigger and bigger. Part of the reason may be organic: the hypothalamus, which regulates appetite, may have been damaged from the head injury. There's an emotional aspect as well—especially if the patient had had weight problems in the past.

WINNING PLAY: If the problem is organic, seek out professional help. If it's an emotional reaction, remove the food from your kitchen. Offer alternate distractions. Your loved one won't think so much about eating if he's busy swimming or gardening or sewing.

Brainteaser # 2: Agitation, Outbursts, and Temper Tantrums

Your husband constantly paces his room. Your wife keeps jumping up from her bed. Your son tells you that you're fat and ugly. Your daughter screams curses at the top of her lungs. None of this behavior is unusual. As we have seen in previous chapters, head injury can cause disinhibition. Emotionally, your loved one will probably be less patient. He will be confused and troubled. He will be anxious and unable to focus on social skills. It may just be a phase, but be prepared for the possibility that he'll have a more volatile personality for the rest of his life. Fortunately, head-injured survivors don't always remember their outbursts. A violent temper flare-up is often over quickly; typically it wasn't the result of deep-seated hostility.

WINNING PLAYS: Be calm and structure your routines. Your agitated loved one needs to feel secure. Ignore outbursts—and warn friends and families when they come to call. Redirect your angry loved one to another topic or goal.

Brainteaser # 3: Depression

It's very common—but it's not fun. However, take heart. Your loved one's morose behavior, his lack of interest in life, his excessive sleeping—all may be signs of progress. He is no longer denying his deficits, and he has begun the slow road to recovery and acceptance. Some other symptoms include:

- Passivity
- Excessive television watching
- Loss of ability to feel pleasure

WINNING PLAYS: If you feel your loved one is acting suicidal in any way, notify a doctor immediately. Try to divert her—enlist her in a game or a walk in the fresh air. Don't blame yourself. It's not your fault. Continue to be pleasant. Ask your physician about the possible use of antidepressant medication. Eventually, the depression may lift and make room for acceptance.

Brainteaser # 4: Increased or Decreased Sexuality

Sexuality, an uncomfortable topic for discussion even in the best of circumstances, can be particularly painful where head-injury is involved because of all the corollary problems: possible loss of love, role reversal, and the physical differences in your sexual partner. With head injury, increased or decreased sexuality is usually a result of hormonal damage in the brain. Sexual hyperactivity is a part of

HEADLINERS

Sunday, December 3, 1989
  "When Dad came to get me I came downstairs and fixed my own breakfast (cornflakes—1 ½ bowls). Then we watched TV while Daddy was working on a carving of a runner. Mom came down around 10:00. We talked about how many more days until I get to come home to stay. I realized it wasn't that much longer (9 days!) We went upstairs to get dressed and I decided I wanted to put my stamps from Turkey and Germany in my stamp book. I ended up putting 2 of the six packets in the book through the day. About 5:00 Daddy, Colleen, and I went out shopping (Pik & Save) and to pick up some pizza for dinner. I also looked through my photo album and could really see how much I'd improved since I'd had my accident."
From a memory book entry written by a RIOSA patient with her parents help to compensate for short-term memory loss. Looking through it later, she would remember her day

disinhibition, the loss of that "civilized" social censor that keeps all of us on a reasonably even keel.

WINNING PLAYS: If your spouse is no longer interested, make sure he's always well-groomed and dressed. If he feels good about himself, he might reassert his sexuality. If he's hyperactive, you probably won't want to go anywhere with him—which can lead to social withdrawal and depression for you both. Instead of hiding, find a support group for him where his behavior can be pointed out. An outpatient rehabilitation program can also be of help. Further, examine your own feelings and needs. Are you afraid sex will further damage your loved one? Are you afraid that the head injury will prevent you from having children? Remember the adage we mentioned at the beginning of this chapter:

ASK QUESTIONS!!!

Brainteaser # 5: Lack of Motivation

It's hard to get going when you are confused, depressed, or overwhelmed. But it's equally hard to listen when the person you love tells you, "I don't want to go to the beach...I don't want to eat dinner...I don't want to help you fold laundry...I don't want to do anything but lie here on the couch and watch reruns of *The Patty Duke Show*." It's at times like these that you must remember your loved one is anxious and sad. Be patient.

WINNING PLAYS: You should have a scheduled routine for each day that includes both definite activities and rest periods. Remember that your loved one needs structure, consistency and repitition in each of their days.

Brainteaser # 6: Dependency

This is a hard one—especially for mothers. It's so easy to fall back into a nurturing role, even if your child is an adult. But this can foster dependency, which will prevent your loved one from growing. The more dependent he becomes, the less responsibility he'll take on. Think of it. You'll have to make all his dentist appointments. You'll always have to do the food shopping. Your social sphere will become smaller. Like the baby in *Who Framed Roger Rabbit?*, you could have a whining, spoiled, cigar-smoking, sexually promiscuous "baby" on your hands.

WINNING PLAYS: Stop yourself before you do for him. Let him cut his own meat. Let him call the drugstore to renew a prescription. Take him shopping with you—or when you make a social call. Have him join a support group where he can make new friends.

These are just a few of the "brainteasers" you might be forced to play. But remember: take care of yourself. And keep a sense of humor. No, life isn't easy. It's full of surprises—and tragedy. But tragedy doesn't have to beget tragedy. You too can start that slow climb up; you too can recover from your loved one's head injury and begin a new life.

Our journey is almost at an end, but to help you even further, we've included some of the most common questions people ask us. Join us for one last chapter....

TWELVE

QUESTIONS FAMILY
MEMBERS COMMONLY ASK

"Beyond the bright searchlights of science,
Out of sight of the windows of sense,
Old Riddles still bid us defiance,
Old questions of Why and of Whence."
—William Cecil Dampier-Whetham (1867–1952),
The Recent Development of Physical Science

Now that we've covered the different aspects of head injury—the hopes, goals, and feelings of family and patient alike—you might be ready to ask some questions of your own.

Unfortunately, we can't stand next to you as you read this book, but we can do the next best thing: answer classic questions that have popped up time and time again in our years of clinical experience. We hope the answers help you as much as they have helped those who first asked....

1. Will my loved one ever be the same?
This is a hard one, because the answer is tough: no. But can your loved one improve? Absolutely, yes. Good therapy, proper rehabilitation, and a positive environment can go far in helping your loved one realize his potential.

One of our patients had a severe head injury when he was run over by a car while leaving work late one afternoon. His wife refused to believe that he would not come out of his injury intact, that he would be different from the man she had married. But the more she denied his injuries, the less help she could give—to her husband and to herself.

123

The trauma happened so fast. You saw the "miracle" of your loved one coming out of a coma. You saw him begin to walk and speak. Why wouldn't you believe that eventually his cognitive abilities would also completely return...

But you can't turn the clock back. What is, is. Instead of running from specialist to specialist looking for another "miracle," you must accept this new reality. With *realistic* hope, both you and your loved one will lead healthier and happier lives.

2. *How long will the healing process take?*

One of the more frustrating aspects of head injury for families is the "wait and see' answers doctors give. These statements really aren't meant as brush-offs. Nor are they meant to be condescending. They are, unfortunately, very honest answers. The fact is, we often don't know how long the healing process will take. Everyone is unique, and predictors can only tell us so much. Even mildly head-injured survivors can take from three to six months to improve. More severe cases need much more time than that. Healing takes time. As with broken arms and broken hearts, mending cannot be rushed.

3. *Can't the doctor make the person I love wake up from a coma?*

No. There is no magic or prince's kiss that can make a coma disappear. Although drugs may be administered while the patient is in a coma, they are usually given to prevent seizures or spasticity—not to help the person awaken. (However, there is active research on drugs that might enhance emergence from coma.) Outside stimulation may not work, but it can't hurt. To this end, family members are encouraged to talk to the patient, hug or stroke him, show him photographs—in short, treat him as if he were awake. As you saw in Chapter Ten, this is rehabilitation—and it can't start soon enough.

4. *Do people in comas feel pain?*

Think of a person in a coma as being under anesthesia for an operation. She might groan or move her body in reaction to a cramp or a cringe, but she'll have no memory of that pain. And, unfortunately, some painful procedures cannot be avoided for patients in a coma. Tracheotomy tubes, nastrogastric tubes, IVs, and catheters must sometimes be inserted—and this foreign apparatus can look especially painful to family members who have never seen any of it before.

5. My loved one's CT scan was normal. Why is he in a coma?

As we have seen in Part I of this book, microscopic damage is not always picked up by CT scans, X rays, or even the more sensitive MRIs. The patient may have diffuse axonal injury or brainstem damage that cannot be seen on the scans but keeps the patient in a coma.

6. Is my loved one malingering?

It's been our experience that most head-injured patients actually try to *minimize* their deficits. However, if your loved one is dramatically acting out, throwing temper tantrums, and screaming, its possible she is suffering from secondary psychological symptoms—in which case you should seek the advice of a head-injury rehab professional. In the meantime, try a reward system such as the one described in Chapter Ten. Find enjoyable activities that you and she can share. Have her join a support group where she can meet others in similar situations. Be patient.

7. Does my loved one have to take her seizure medicine forever?

Probably not—but don't underestimate its importance: Seizures can cause additional physical injury. Antiseizure medicine should be monitored: it's possible that its side effects might interfere with your loved one's cognitive retraining. It's important to note that antiseizure medicine should never just be stopped suddenly; abrupt withdrawal may actually *cause* seizures. Instead, the medication should be tapered off slowly—under a doctor's full supervision.

8. How do I know when I need help?

Unfortunately, we can be so intent on aiding those we love that we neglect ourselves. If you become overstressed, you may be:

- Unable to sleep
- Poorly groomed
- Overwhelmed with guilt or feelings of unworthiness
- Feeling totally isolated and alone, with nowhere to turn

- Starting to use alcohol or drugs excessively
- Stricken with a sense of hopelessness—for yourself and the person you love

Remember, you must take care of yourself before you can take care of anyone else. If you are experiencing any of these symptoms, speak to your case manager—and seek out professional therapeutic help.

9. What about experimental therapies? Do they work?

Here's the rundown on some of the more popular fads:

- *Vitamins.* There is absolutely no evidence to support the use of vitamin megadoses. If your head-injured loved one is being given a nutritional supplement, it will contain all the vitamins he needs.

- *Special Diets.* Unfortunately, there's no such thing as "brain food." Nor is there any evidence that hair or nail testing is useful in diagnosing deficiencies in trace elements and/or minerals.

- *Hyperbaric Oxygen.* It's been tried for central nervous system diseases such as multiple sclerosis, but without success. It doesn't work for MS, it won't work for head injuries, either.

- *Brain Implants.* Although there has been experimental research on brain implants for patients with Parkinson's disease, the topic is very controversial. Favorite sci-fi flicks aside, there is absolutely no clinical evidence that implants could improve cognitive function or memory.

- *Electric Therapy/Magnetotherapy.* Using electricity or magnetic fields to stimulate the skull does not improve anything—least of all cognitive function.

- *Acupuncture.* Yes, it does work to control pain, but acupuncture has yet to be proved an effective treatment for memory loss or cognitive dysfunction. Nor has it been proven to help spasticity, paralysis, or motor function.

- *Chelation Therapy.* This is a process that uses chemicals to remove minerals, metals, and trace elements from the body. However, it's an unproved approach that could be dangerous. It's not performed by any reputable physician, nor is it supported by any recognized scientific organization.

- *Herbal Medicine.* Folk healers have long used herbs and roots to treat a variety of medical disorders. But curing

HEADLINERS

THE PRIME OF MR. JAMES BRADY

It was a tragedy—it almost seemed as if history were repeating itself much too soon. Then-President Reagan had been shot, but it was his up-and-coming Press Secretary who took the brunt of the would-be assassin's bullet. That was in 1980. One and a half years later, Brady had made vast improvement. Having escaped death from brain swelling and fluid build-up, Mr. Brady was already able to get around in a wheelchair. He could make jokes. Even his political acumen was intact. Why? Perhaps it was because he had such a strong personality. Perhaps it was the tremendous support he received. Perhaps it was his motivation to succeed in rehabilitation....

Today, James Brady is no longer a President's press secretary. But he holds a key political role—National Honorary Chairperson of the National Head Injury Foundation—and is a role model and source of inspiration for thousands of head-injured patients across the world.

constipation or migraines is one thing. Developing memory, improving cognitive function, and changing inappropriate behavior are activities best managed by rehabilitation specialists.

Although herbalist "rainmakers" might seem appealing, a hopeful beacon of light in a life that seems closed in darkness, there is no scientific evidence to support their sometimes extravagant claims. Unfortunately, there are no miracles—rehabilitation is a slow, steady process.

10. My child was injured over a year ago—and the stress has been enormous. My family is falling apart. Where can we go for some solid help?

The non-profit National Head Injury Foundation (NHIF) has over 44 state associations and affiliates, plus over 375 support groups across the nation. They also have a directory that lists over 400 rehabilitation hospitals from coast to coast. The NHIF also sponsors conferences, and has a wide range of research resources you can receive by mail. To speak to a *real* person and to receive *real* help, call their hotline: 1-800-444-NHIF.

Our book is coming to an end; our time together is almost over. We hope these questions were some of the ones you yourself had been wanting to ask, or at least that they've given you food for thought. We know there's plenty on your mind.

EPILOGUE:
THE FUTURE IS NOW

We firmly believe that head injury, while traumatic, is not the worst thing that could happen. If one of our children was in a terrible accident, we would want to do everything possible to save him or her. We would want the emergency and intensive-care units to do everything they could to keep our child alive. We would rather have this child in a wheelchair for the rest of his or her life, relearning new behaviors, discovering old memories, and finding new cognitive skills and activities of daily life, than gone from our lives forever.

The motto of the National Head Injury Foundation is "Because life after head injury may never be the same." But it *is* life. It hasn't ended.

And that life can still be rewarding. It can still be dignified. It can still be hopeful. Long-term success is possible. At RIOSA, we see proof of this every single day.

A head-injured person wrote these words in a National Head Injury Foundation article: "One friend who told me that 75 percent of me was better than 100 percent of others she knew, will never know how much she helped me."

It is our hope that this book has helped you. We hope you now have a better understanding of head injury—its symptoms and its pain. We hope you feel you've had a short course in the rehabilitation process—that you now know and understand how head-injury rehabilitation works, and why. We hope we have given you some confidence, some "essence," that you can take away and that will keep you strong and accepting.

We hope we have helped you to find hope—and a reason to go on.

That is success. And it's what head-injury rehabilitation is all about—the success of helping others. In fact, that's probably what life itself is all about....

EDUCATIONAL SOURCES

American Occupational Therapy Association
1383 Piccard Drive
Box 1725
Rockville, MD 20850-4375
(301) 948-9626

American Physical Therapy Association
1111 North Fairfax Street
Alexandria, VA 22314
1-800-999-2782

American Speech-Language-Hearing Association
10801 Rockville Pike
Rockville, Maryland 20852
(301) 897-5700 (Voice or TTY)

Association for Children and Adults with Learning
Disabilities
Literary Depository
4156 Library Road
Pittsburgh, Pennsylvania 15234
(412) 341-1515

Association for Persons with Severe Handicaps
7010 Roosevelt Way NE
Seattle, WA 98115
(206) 523-8446

Association of Rehabilitation Nurses
2506 Gross Point Road
Evanston, IL 60201
(312) 475-1000

Commission on Accreditation of Rehab Facilities (CARF)
101 N. Wilmot Road, Suite 500
Tucson, Arizona 85711
(602) 748-1212

JCAHO (Joint Commission on Accreditation of Hospital
Organizations)
One Renaissance Boulevard
Oakbrook Terrace, Illinois 60181
(708) 916-5600

Joseph P. Kennedy, Jr. Foundation
1350 New York Avenue, N.W.
Suite 500
Washington, DC. 20005-4709
(202) 393-1250

The Moody Foundation
704 Moody National Bank Building
Galveston, Texas 77550
(409) 763-5333

National Head Injury Foundation, Inc.
333 Turnpike Road
Southboro, MA 01772
1-800-444-NHIF

Rehab Hospital Services Corporation (RHSC)
1010 Wisconsin Ave., N.W.
Washington, D.C. 20007

Rehabilitation Institute of San Antonio (RIOSA)
9119 Cinnamon Hill
San Antonio, Texas 78240
(512) 691-0737

U.S. Government Printing Office
Superintendent of Documents
Washington, D.C. 20402
(202) 783-3238
Directory of Living Aids for the Disabled Person

SOURCES

Alexander, Michael P., M.D., "Neurobehavioral Consequences of Closed Head Injury," *Neurology and Neurosurgery (Update Series)*, 5:20, 1984.

Alves, Wayne M., Ph.D., and John A. Jane, M.D., Ph.D., "Mild Brain Injury: Damage and Outcome." IN: *Central Nervous System Status Report*, edited by D. Becker, M.D., and J. Povlishock, Ph.D., National Institute of Health, Bethesda, MD, 1985. Reprinted by National Head Injury Foundation, Inc., Southborough, MA: Article #85-021.

Barrer, Andrew E., Ph.D., and Douglas H. Ruben, M.A., "Understanding the Etiology of Brain Injury." Excerpted from *Readings in Brain Injury*, edited by Andrew E. Barrer, Ph.D., and Douglas H. Ruben, M.A. Reprinted by National Head Injury Foundation, Inc., Southborough, MA: Article #B1084.

Barry, Philip, "A Psychological Perspective of Acute Brain Injury Rehabilitation," *Cognitive Rehabilitation*, 4:4, July-August 1986, pp. 18–21.

Batson, Meg, M.A., "Alcohol & TBI: A Problematic Pair," *Headlines: The Brain Injury Magazine from New Medico Head Injury System*, 1:1, Spring 1990.

Ben-Yishay, Yehuda, Ph.d., "The Role of Clinical Neuropsychology in Diagnosis and Rehabilitation." IN: *Head Injury: Help, Hope & Information*, 3rd ed. Albany, N.Y.: The New York State Head Injury Association, Inc., 1984.

———, and George Prigatano, Ph.D., "Chapter 27: Cognitive Remediation." In: *Rehabilitation of the Adult and Child with Traumatic Brain Injury*, 2nd ed., edited by Mitchell Rosenthal, Ph.D., Ernest R. Griffith, M.D., and Michael R. Bond, M.D. Philadelphia: F.A. Davis Company, 1990.

Berrol, Sheldon, M.D., "Issues in Cognitive Rehabilitation," *Archives of Neurology,* vol. 47, February 1990.

———, "Issues of Sexuality in Head-Injured Adults." In: *Sexuality and Physical Disability,* edited by David G. Bullard and Susan E. Knight. St. Louis: C.V. Mosby Co., 1981. Reprinted by National Head Injury Foundation, Inc., Southborough, MA: Article #81-010.

Binder, L.M., and J. Rattock, "Assessment of the Post-Concussive Syndrome After Mild Head Trauma." In: *Assessment of the Behavioral Consequences of Head Trauma,* edited by M.D. Lezak. New York: Alan R. Liss, Inc., 1989, pp. 37–48.

Blackerby, W.F., Ph.D., "Disruption of Sexuality Following Head Injury," lecture handout materials.

———, *Head Injury Rehabilitation: Sexuality After TBI,* HDI Professional Series on Traumatic Brain Injury no. 10, edited by William H. Burke, Ph.D., Michael D. Wesolowski, Ph.D., and William F. Blackerby, III, Ph.D. Houston, Texas: HDI Publishers, 1988.

———, "Disruption of Sexuality Can Have Traumatic Effect." Reprinted by National Head Injury Foundation, Inc., Southborough, MA: Article #87-001.

Bond, M., "The Psychiatry of Closed Head Injury." In: *Closed Head Injury: Psychological, Social and Family Consequences,* edited by N. Brooks. Oxford, England: Oxford University Press, 1984, pp. 148–78.

Bond, Michael R., M.D., Ph.D., "Psychobehavioral Consequences of Severe Brain Injury," *Trends in Rehabilitation,* Byron Mawr Rehabilitation Hospital Quarterly Magazine, Summer 1986. Reprinted by National Head Injury Foundation, Inc., Southborough, MA: Article #86-002.

Brigman, Cynthia, Carol Dickey, and Louise J. Zegeer, "Agitated, Aggressive, Patient," *American Journal of Nursing,* 83:10, October 1983. Reprinted in *Readings in Brain Injury,* edited by Andrew E. Barrer, Ph.D., and Douglas H. Ruben, M.A. Guilford, Conn.: Special Learning Corporation, 1984.

Brooks, D. Neil, Ph.D., "Chapter 12: Cognitive Deficits." In: *Rehabilitation of the Adult and Child with Traumatic Brain Injury,* 2nd ed., edited by Mitchell Rosenthal, Ph.d., Ernest R. Griffith, M.D., and Michael R. Bond, M.D. Philadelphia: F.A. Davis Company, 1990.

Burke, Michael, "Reflections of a Brother," *Cognitive Rehabilitation,* 2:3, May-June 1984. Reprinted by National Head Injury Foundation, Inc., Southborough, MA: First Person Packet #P-007.

Burke, William H., with Mark Guth, Richard Guare, and Michael D. Wesolowski, *Head Injury Rehabilitation: An Overview,* HDI Professional Series on Traumatic Brain Injury no. 1, edited by William H. Burke, Ph.D., Michael D. Wesolowski, Ph.D., and William F. Blackerby, III, Ph.D. Houston, Texas: HDI Publishers, 1988.

————, with Michael D. Wesolowski, *Head Injury Rehabilitation: Applied Behavior Analysis in Head Injury Rehab,* HDI Professional Series on Traumatic Brain Injury no. 2, edited by William H. Burke, Ph.D., Michael D. Wesolowski Ph. D., and William F. Blackerby, II, Ph.D. Houston, Texas: HDI Publishers, 1988.

————, with Richard J. Zawlocki, Michael D. Wesolowski, and Mark L. Guth, *Head Injury Rehabilitation: Developing Social Skills,,* the HDI Professional Series on Traumatic Brain Injury no. 9, edited by William H. Burke, Ph.D., Michael D. Wesolowski, Ph.D., and William F. Blackerby, III, Ph.D. Houston, Texas: HDI Publishers, 1988.

Butler, Robert W., Ph.D., and Norman S. Namerow, M.D., "Cognitive Retraining in Brain-Injury Rehabilitation: A Critical Review," *Journal of Neurological Rehabilitation,* 2:3, 1988.

Byrne, Robert, *1,911 Best Things Anybody Ever Said.* New York: Fawcett Columbine, 1988.

Chance, Paul, "Life After head Injury," *Psychology Today,* October 1986. Reprinted by National Head Injury Foundation, Inc., Southborough, MA: Article #86-022.

Cytowic, Richard E., "The Long Ordeal of James Brady," *The New York Times Magazine,* 131:7, September 1981. Reprinted in *Readings in Brain Injury,* edited by Andrew E. Barrer, Ph.D., and Douglas H. Ruben, M.A. Guilford, Conn.: Special Learning Corporation, 1984.

Davis, Diana L., Ph.D., *Manifestations of Neuropsychological Deficits Examples.* Austin, Texas: Healthcare Rehabilitation Center, lecture handout.

Deaton, Ann V., Ph.D., *Pediatric Head Trauma: A Guide for Families,* Cumberland Hospital, New Kent, Virginia. Austin, Texas. Healthcare International, Inc., 1987.

DiGiuseppi, Carolyn, M.D., M.P.H., Frederick P. Rivara, M.D., M.P.H., Thomas D. Koepsell, M.D., M.P.H., and Lincoln Polissar, Ph.D., "Bicycle Helmet Use by Children: Evaluation of a Community-Wide Helmet Campaign," *Journal of the American Medical Association,* 262:16, October 27, 1989.

Dobkin, B.R., "Head Trauma," *New York Times Magazine,* October 9, 1988, pp. 50–51.

Eisenberg, Howard M., M.D. "Outcome After Head Injury: General Considerations and Neurobehavioral Recovery, Part I: General Considerations." In: *Central Nervous System Trauma Status Report, 1985,* edited by D. Becker, M.D., and J. Povlishock, Ph.D., National Institute of Health, Bethesda, MD. Reprinted by National Head Injury Foundation, Inc., Southborough, MA: Article #85-025.

Feld, Karen, "How Doctors Treat Severe Head Injury," *Parade Magazine,* March 18, 1984. Reprinted in *Readings in Brain Injury,* edited by Anderw E. Barrer, Ph.D., and Douglas H. Ruben, M.A. Guilford, Conn.: Special Learning Corporation, 1984.

Fisher, Jerid M., Ph.D., "Cognitive and Behavioral Consequences of Closed Head Injury," *Seminars in Neurology,* 5:3, September 1985. Reprinted by National Head Injury Foundation, Inc., Southborough, MA: Article #85-010.

Fordyce, David J., James R. Roueche, and George P. Prigatano, "Enhanced Emotional Reactions in Chronic Head Trauma Patients," *Journal of Neurology, Neurosurgery, and Psychiatry,* vol. 46, 1983.

Fralish, Kathleen, Ph.D., "Characteristics of Persons with Head Injury." In: *Innovations in Head Injury Rehabilitation,* edited by Paul M. Deustch, Ph.D., and Kathleen B. Fralish, Ph.D. New York, N.Y.: Matthew Bender, 1988.

Frankowski, Ralph F., Ph.D., John F. Anegers, Ph.D., and Steven Whitman, Ph.D., "Epidemiological and Descriptive Studies, Part I: The Descriptive Epidemiology of Head Trauma in the United States." In *Central Nervous System Trauma Report,* reprinted by National Head Injury Foundation, Inc., Southborough, MA: Article #85-019.

Fryer, Jeanne, Ph.D., and Kathleen Fralish, Ph.D., "Cognitive Rehabilitation." In: *Innovations in Head Injury Rehabilitation,* edited by Paul M. Deustch, Ph.D., and Kathleen B. Fralish, Ph.D. New York, N.Y.: Matthew Bender, 1988.

Furst, Charles, Ph.D., "The Neuropsychological Evaluation." Excerpted from *Head Injury Symptoms: Brain Damage vs. Neurosis,* Los Angeles Trial Lawyers Association, 1984. Reprinted by National Head Injury Foundation, Inc., Southborough, MA: Article #BO484.

Goldberg, Stephen, M.D., *Clinical Neuroanatomy Made Riduculously Simple.* Miami, Fla: MedMaster, Inc., 1979.

Goldstein, Felicia C., and Harvey S. Levin, "Epidemiology of Pediatric Closed Head Injury: Incidence, Clincal Characteristics, and Risk Factors," *Journal of Learning Disabilities,* 20:9, November 1987. Reprinted by National Head Injury Foundation, Inc., Southborough, MA: Article #87-041.

Grafman, Jordan H., Ph.D., "Cognitive and Behavioral Sequelae of Head Injury," *Recent Advances in Head Injury: Annual Course #420,* American Academy of Neurology, Wednesday, April 19, 1989.

Guare, Richard, with Molly Samson, Mark Guth, Susie Warren, and William H. Burke, *Head Injury Rehabilitation: Developing the TBI Rehab Plan,* HDI Professional Series on Traumatic Brain Injury no. 4, edited by William H. Burke, Ph.D., Michael D. Wesolowski, Ph.D., and William F. Blackerby, III, Ph.D. Houston, Texas: HDI Publishers, 1988.

Harvey E. Jacobs, Ph.D., "Chapter 20: Adult Community Integration." In: *Traumatic Brain Injury (Comprehensic Neurologic Rehabilitation),* vol. 2, edited by P. Bachyrita. New York: Demos Publications, 1989, p. 331.

Hawley, Lenore A., *A Family Guide to the Rehabilitation of the Severely Head-Injured Patient.* Austin, Texas: Healthcare International, Inc., 1984, 1987.

HDI Professional Series on Traumatic Brain Injury, no. 8, edited by William H. Burke, Ph.D., Michael D. Wesolowski, Ph.D., and William F. Blackerby, III, Ph.D. Houston, Texas: HDI Publishers, 1988.

Hoine, Haskel, Ph.D., "Behavior Management of the Agitated, Aggressive Head Injured Patient," *Progress Report,* Rehabilitation Institute of San Antonio, Winter 1990.

———, "Psychological Adjustment to Disability," *Progress Report,* Rehabilitation Institute of San Antonio, Fall 1989.

Hopewell, C. Alan, *Head Injury Rehabilitation: Adaptive Driving After TBI,* HDI Professional Series on Traumatic Brain Injury no. 5, edited by William H. Burke, Ph.D., Michael D. Wesolowski, Ph.D., and William F. Blackerby, III, Ph.D. Houston, Texas: HDI Publishers, 1988.

———, "Practical Treatment Methods for Emotional Dysfunction," lecture handout.

Howard, Michael E., Ph.D., "Family Adjustment to Head Injury," lecture handout.

———, "Outcome from Head Injury," *Family Handbook of Head Injury,* lecture handout.

———, "Recovery from Head Trauma by Levels of Cognitive Functioning," *Family Handbook of Head Injury,* lecture handout.

Hutchison, Ruth, M.S., and Terry Hutchison, M.D., Ph.D.,

in collaboration with members of the Texas Head Injury Foundation, *Head Injury: A Booklet for Families*. Texas: The Texas Head Injury Foundation, 1983.

Kasowski, Janice Cortis, "Silent Epidemic," *First Person Accounts*. Reprinted by National Head Injury Foundation, Inc., Southborough, MA: Article #P-007.

Kline, Jeanette, "Knowing *What Was* Made It Difficult to Accept *What Is*," *First Person Accounts*. Printed by National Head Injury Foundation, Inc., Southborough, MA: Article #P-007.

Klonoff, Pamela, Ph.D., Kevin P O'Brien, Ph.D., George P. Prigatano, Ph.D., Dennis A. Chiapello, M.S., C.C.C. -S.L.P., and Marie Cunningham, C.T.R.S./C.R.T., "Cognitive Retraining After Traumatic Brain Injury and Its Role in Facilitating Awareness," *Journal of Head Trauma Rehabilitation*, 4:3, 1989.

Kraus, Jess F., Mary Ann Black, Nancy Hessol, Pacita Ley, William Rokaw, Constance Sullivan, Sharon Bowers, Sharen Knowlton, and Lawrence Marshall, "The Incidence of Acute Brain Injury and Serious Impairment in a Defined Population," *American Journal of Epidemiology*, 119:2, 1984. Reprinted by National Head Injury Foundation, Inc., Southborough, MA: Article #84-026.

Levin, Harvey S., Ph.D., and Howard M. Eisenberg, M.D., "Postconcussional Syndrome," *Neurotrauma Medical Report*, 2:4, Fall 1988.

Lewis, Frank, Ph.D., *Head Injury Rehabilitation: Developing Adaptive Work Behaviors*, HDI Professional Series on Traumatic Brain Injury no. 17, edited by William H. Burke, Ph.D., Michael D. Wesolowski, Ph.D., and William F. Blackerby, III, Ph.D. Houston, Texas: HDI Publishers, 1988.

Lezak, Muriel D., Ph.D., "Living with the Characterologically Altered Brain Injured Patient," *Journal of Clinical Psychiatry*, 1978. Reprinted by the National Head Injury Foundation, Inc., Southborough, MA: Article #78-001.

Livingston, M.G., M.D. "Chapter 16: Effects on the Family System." In: *Rehabilitation of the Adult and Child with Traumatic Brain Injury*, 2nd ed., edited by Mitchell Rosenthal, Ph.D., Ernest R. Griffith, M.D., and Michael R. Bond, M.D. Philadelphia: F.A. Davis Company, 1990.

Livingston, Martin G., M.D. M.R.C. Psych., and D. Neil Brooks, Ph.D., "The Burden on Families of the Brain Injured: A Review," *Journal of Head Trauma Rehabilitation*, 3:4, December 1988.

Lynch, William J., Ph.D., "Chapter 22: Neuropsychological

Assessment." In: *Rehabilitation of the Adult and Child with Traumatic Brain Injury,* 2nd ed., edited by Mitchell Rosenthal, Ph.D., Ernest R. Griffith, M.D., and Michael R. Bond, M.D. Philadelphia: F.A. Davis Company, 1990.

McMahon, B.T., and Flowers, S.M., "The High Cost of a Bump on the Head," *Business and Health,* vol: 3, June 1986, pp. 7–8.

Miller, J. Douglas, M.D., Ph.D., and Patricia A. Jones, Dip. Phys., M.Sc., "Chapter 17: Minor Head Injury." In: *Rehabilitation of the Adult and Child with Traumatic Brain Injury,* 2nd ed., edited by Mitchell Rosenthal, Ph.D., Ernest R. Griffith, M.D., and Michael R. Bond, M.D. Philadelphia: F.A. Davis Company, 1990.

Mishkin, David, Ph.D., and Elizabeth Kampe, M.A., "Guidelines for the Management of Common Behavioral Problems With Post Trauma Patients." Reprinted by National Head Injury Foundation, Inc., Southborough, MA: Article #83-014.

Namerow, Norman S., M.D., *Cognitive and Behavioral Aspects of Brain Injury Rehabilitation,* Neurological Clinics, 5:4, 1987, pp. 569–83.

National Head Injury Foundation, *About Head Injuries.* South Deerfield, MA: A Scriptographic Booklet by Channing L. Bete Co., Inc., 1987.

National Head Injury Foundation, Inc., *Brochure,* National Head Injury Foundation, Inc., 333 Turnpike Road, Southborough, MA 01722.

National Head Injury Foundation, Inc., *Newsletter,* volume 9, nos. 3 and 4, Winter 1989–90.

National Head Injury Foundation, Inc., "Questions About Traumatic Brain Injury (TBI)," 1988. Article #84-005.

New York State Head Injury Association, Inc. "Head Injury Facts and Figures, General Characteristics." In: *Head Injury: Help, Hope & Information: A Family Guide,* 3rd ed. Albany, N.Y.: New York State Head Injury Association, Inc., 1984.

Oddy, Michael, and Michael Humphrey, "Social Recovery During the Year Following Severe Head Injury," *Journal of Neurology, Neurosurgery, and Psychiatry,* vol. 43, 1980.

Peterman, Bill, "A Substance Abuse Program for Head Injury Survivors." Reprinted by National Head Injury Foundation, Inc., Southborough, MA: Article #86-028.

Phoebus, Brenda, M.A., C.C.C./S.L.P., "Coma Stimulation: The Role of the Speech Pathologist," *Journal of Audiology and Speech Pathology,* 14:2, Fall/Winter 1988.

Pollack, I.W., "Chapter 5: Traumatic Brain Injury," In:

Neuropsychological Treatment After Brain Injury, edited by D.W. Ellis and A.L. Christensen. Kluwer Academic Publishers, Norwell, MA: 1989, p. 420.

Prigatano, George P., "Emotion and Motivation in Recovery and Adaptation after Brain Damage," *Psychiatric Medicine,* 7:1, 1989.

———, "Psychiatric Aspects of Head Injury: Problem Areas and Suggested Guidelines for Research." In: *Neurobehavioral Recovery from Head Injury.* New York: Oxford University Press, 1987.

———, "Rehabilitation Interventions After Traumatic Brain Injury," *BNI Quarterly,* 4:2, Spring 1988.

———, and others, *Neuropsychological Rehabilitation after Brain Injury.* The Johns Hopkins University Press, Baltimore/London, 1985, p. 63.

———, David J. Fordyce, Harriet K. Zeiner, James R. Roueche, Mary Pepping, Beth Case Wood, "Neuropsychological Rehabilitation After Closed Head Injury in Young Adults," *Journal of Neurology, Neurosurgery, and Psychiatry,* vol. 47, 1984.

———, Mary Pepping, and Pamela Klonoff, "Chapter Seven: Cognitive, Personality, and Psychosocial Factors in the Neuropsychological Assessment of Brain-Injured Patients." In: *Clinical Neuropsychology of Intervention,* edited by Uzzell and Gross, Norwell, MA: Martinus Nijhoff Publishing, 1986.

———, Monte L. Stahl, William C. Orr, and Harriet K. Zeiner, "Sleep and Dreaming Disturbances in Closed Head Injury Patients," *Journal of Neurology, Neurosurgery, and Psychiatry,* vol. 45, 1982.

———, Kevin P. O'Brien, Ph.d., and Pamela S. Klonoff, Ph.D., "The Clinical Management of Paranoid Delusions in Postacute Traumatic Brain-Injured Patients," *Head Trauma Rehabilitation, 3:3, 1988.*

Restak, Richard M., M.D., *The Brain.* New York: Bantam Books, 1984.

Rimel, Rebecca, W. R.N., N.P., John A. Jane, M.D. Ph.D., and Michael R. Bond, M.D., Ph.D., "Chapter Two: Characteristics of the Head-Injured Patient." In: *Rehabilitation of the Adult and Child with Traumatic Brain Injury,* 2nd ed., edited by Mitchell Rosenthal, Ph.D., Ernest R. Griffith, M.D., and Michael R. Bond, M.D. Philadelphia: F.A. Davis Company, 1990.

Rosenthal, Mitchell, Ph.D., and Michael R. Bond, M.D., Ph.D., "Chapter 13: "Behavioral and Psychiatric Sequelae." In: *Rehabilitation of the Adult and Child with Traumatic*

Brain Injury, 2nd ed., edited by Mitchell Rosenthal, Ph.D., Ernest R. Griffith, M.D., and Michael R. Bond, M.D., Philadelphia: F.A. Davis Company, 1990.

Sachs, Paul R., Ph.D., "Grief and the Traumatically Head-Injured Adult," *Rehabilitation Nursing,* 9:1, January/February 1984. Reprinted by National Head Injury Foundation, Inc., Southborough, MA: Article #84-031.

Salazar, Andres, M.D., "Neurologic Sequelae of Closed and Penetrating Head Injury," *Recent Advances in Head Injury: Annual Course #420,* American Academy of Neurology, Wednesday, April 19, 1989.

Senelick, Richard C., M.D., "Head Injury: A Primer," *Progress Report,* Rehabilitation Institute of San Antonio, Winter 1990.

———, "Mild Head Injury: Separating the Wheat From the Chaff," Beau County Medical Journal, TK.

———, "The Growth of Rehabilitation: Why RIOSA Stands Out," *Progress Report,* Rehabilitation Institute of San Antonio, Fall 1989.

———, "The Use of Medications in the Head Injured Patient," *Progress Report,* Rehabilitation Institute of San Antonio, Spring 1990.

Shapiro, Kenneth, M.D., "Head Injury in Children." In: *Central Nervous System Trauma Status Report,* 1985. Reprinted by National Head Injury Foundation, Inc., Southborough, MA: Article #85-018.

Silver, J.M., S. Yudofsky, and R.E. Hales, "Chapter 10: Neuropsychiatric Aspects of Traumatic Brain Injury." In: *The American Psychiatric Press Textbook of Neuropsychiatry,* edited by Robert E. Hales, M.D., and Stuart C. Yudofsky, M.D. Washington, D.C.: American Psychiatric Press, Inc., 1987, p. 490.

Slaby, Andrew E., Ph.D., M.P.H., *Aftershock: Surviving the Delayed Effects of Trauma, Crisis, and Loss.* New York: Villard Books, 1989.

Tampa General Rehabilitation Center, Tampa, Florida, with Dana S. DeBoskey, Ph.D., and Karen Morin, M.S.W., *Head Injury: A Guide For Families,* HDI Coping Series no. 1. Houston, Texas: HDI Publishers, 1989.

Tampa General Rehabilitation Center, Tampa, Florida, with Dana S. DeBoseky, Ph.D., Tyler Benyo, M.Ed., Connie Calub, M.Ed., Thomas Oleson, M.S., and Karen Morin, M.S.W., *Hiring the Head Injured: What to Expect,* HDI Coping Series no. 3. Houston, Texas: HDI Publishers, 1989.

Tampa General Rehabilitation Center, Tampa, Florida, with

Connie Calub, M.Ed., Dana S. DaBoskey, Ph.D., John Burton, M.S., Cathy Cook, M.S., Lisa Lowe, B.A., Dorothy McHenry, M.A., and Karen Morinn, M.S.W., *Teaching the Head Injured: What to Expect,* HDI Coping Series no. 5, Houston, Texas: HDI Publishers, 1989.

Tampa General Rehabilitation Center, Tampa, Florida, with Dana S. DeBoskey, Ph.D., Connie J. Calub, M.D., John Burton, M.S., and Karen Morin, M.S.W., *Life After Head Injury: Who Am I?,* HDI Coping Series no. 4. Houston, Texas: HDI Publishers, 1989.

Thickman, Mark, P.T., and John D. Ranseen, Ph.D., "Personality Changes Associated with Head Trauma: Implications for Rehabilitation Specialists," *Topics in Acute Care and Trauma Rehabilitation,* Journal Editor, Mary Kay Campbell, B.A., P.T., and "Head Injury" issue edited by Judith Verbanets, M.S., P.T., 1:1, July 1986.

Thompson, Robert S., M.D., Frederick P. Rivara, M.D., M.P.H., and Diane C. Thompson, M.S., "A Case-Control Study of the Effectiveness of Bicycle Safety Helmets," *New England Journal of Medicine,* 320:21, May 25, 1989.

Traphagan, J.W.P., *Advocating for Funds.* Southborough, MA: National Head Injury Foundation, Inc., June 1988.

Traphagan, J.W.P., *Community Re-Entry.* Southborough, MA: National Head Injury Foundation, Inc., April 1988.

Tressler, Lance, ed., *Coma Assessment Scales with Stimulation Techniques,* National Head Injury Foundation, Inc., Article #8406. 1984.

Vogenthaler, Donald R., Ph.D., "An Overview of Head Injury: Its Consequences and Rehabilitation," *Brain Injury,* Jul-Sept 1(1):113–27, 1987.

Volpe, Bruce T., M.D., "Topics in the Rehabilitation of the Head-Injured Patient," lecture handout.

Wasco, James, M.D., "New Hope for Behavior Patients," *Headlines: The Brain Injury Magazine from New Medico Head Injury System,* 1:1, Spring 1990.

Weber, Lynn M., and Judity Verbanets, "Assessing Balance Performance in Moderate Brain Injury," *Topics in Acute Care and Trauma Rehabilitation,* 1:1, July 1986.

Weddell, Rodger, Michael Oddy, and David Jenkins, "Social Adjustment After Rehabilitation: A Two Year Follow-up of Patients with Severe Head Injury," *Psychological Medicine,* vol. 10, 1980.

Weinstein, Amy, with Elizabeth Moes and Margaret O'Connor, *Head Injury Rehabilitation: Management of Memory Disorders,* The HDI Professional Series on Traumatic Brain Injury. Houston, Texas: HDI Publishers, 1988.

Wesolowski, Michael, with Arnie Zencius, Richard J. Zawlocki, and William H. Burke, *Head Injury Rehabilitation: Developing Self-Control,* HDI Professional Series on Traumatic Brain Injury no. 14, edited by William H. Burke, Ph.D., Michael D. Wesolowski, Ph.D., and William F. Blackerby, III, Ph.D. Houston, Texas: HDI Publishers, 1988.

Wesolowski, Michael, with Richard J. Zawlocki, *Head Injury Rehabilitation: Teaching Job Seeking Skills,* HDI Professional Series on Traumatic Brain Injury no. 16, edited by William H. Burke, Ph.D., Michael D. Wesolowski, Ph.D., and William F. Blackerby, III, Ph.D. Houston, Texas: HDI Publishers, 1988.

Williams, Janet, M.S.W., *What to Look for When Selecting a Rehabilitation Facility: A Working Guide.* National Head Injury Foundation, Inc., Southborough, MA: Article #85-011.

Wilson, Amani, Ph.D., *Clinical Applications of Neuropsychological Testing: An Overview.* Wellesley, Mass.: River Bridge Associates. Reprinted by National Head Injury Foundation, Inc., Southborough, MA: Article #B1384.

Wood, R.L., "Chapter 10, *Closed Head Injury: Psychological, Social and Family Consequences.* In: Brooks, N. (ed), New York, Oxford University Press, 1984, pp. 195–220.

Ylvisaker, Mark, *Head Injury Rehabilitation: Head Injury Rehab with Children and Adults,* HDI Professional Series on Traumatic Brain Injury no. 12, edited by William H. Burke, Ph.D., Michael D. Wesolowski, Ph.D., and William F. Blackerby, III, Ph.D. Houston, Texas: HDI Publishers, 1988.

Ylvisaker, Mark, *Head Injury Rehabilitation: Management of Communication and Language Deficits,* HDI Professional Series on Traumatic Brain Injury no. 20, edited by William H. Burke, Ph.D., Michael D. Wesolowski, Ph.D., and William F. Blackerby, III, Ph.D. Houston, Texas: HDI Publishers, 1988.

Zinner, Ellen, Ph.D., "Mother's Grief Reactions Studied," For Your Information column in *Newsletter,* Winter 1989-90, vol. 9, no. 3 & 4, National Head Injury Foundation, Inc. Southborough, MA 01772.

————, "What are the Options?" Compiled from interviews with William Burke, Ph.D., John Fanning, Ph.D., Frank Sparadeo, Ph.D., Allan Kraft, L.M.S.W., Jayne M. Wilson, M.S.W., and Grace Smythe, *Headlines: The Brain Injury Magazine from New Medico Head Injury System,* 1:1, Spring 1990.

————, "Up Close with Case Manager Sue Haley," *Progress Report,* Rehabilitation Institute of San Antonio, Winter 1990.

————, "High Observation Unit," *Progress Report,* Rehabilitation Institute of San Antonio, Winter 1990.

————, "If This is Therapy, Why Are We Having So Much Fun," *Progress Report,* Rehabilitation Institute of San Antonio, Fall 1989.

————, "New Drugs Could Curb Brain Damage," *Headlines: The Brain Injury Magazine from New Medico Head Injury System,* 1:1, Spring 1990.

————, "Nurse Liaison Help Smooth Transitions," *Progress Report,* Rehabilitation Institute of San Antonio, Fall 1989.

————, "Return to Work," *Progress Report,* Rehabilitation Institute of San Antonio, Fall 1989.

————, "Trauma Happens to People: Adjusting to Disability," *Progress Report,* Rehabilitation Institute of San Antonio, Fall 1989.

————, *Some Symptoms and Characteristic Behavior Patterns of Those Who Have Suffered Traumatic Closed Head Injuries,* Institute of Physical Medicine and Rehabilitation, Peoria, Illinois, Reprinted by National Head Injury Foundation, Inc., Southborough, MA: Article #84-007.

————, "Behavior Analysis: Treatment That Works for TBI." Compiled from *Applied Behavior Analysis in Head Injury Rehabilitation* by William Burke, Ph.D., and Michael Wesolowski, Ph.D., in *Rehabilitation Nursing,* 13:4, 1988, and *Headlines: The Brain Injury Magazine from New Medico Head Injury System,* 1:1, Spring 1990.

————, "Coma Intervention Tugs on Heartstrings," *Headlines: The Brain Injury Magazine from New Medico Head Injury System,* 1:1, Spring 1990.

————, "Emotionally Charged," *Headlines: The Brain Injury Magazine from New Medico Head Injury System,* 1:1, Spring 1990.

————, *Co-Treatment Outline,* Rehabilitation Institute of San Antonio, lecture handout.

INDEX

About the Authors

RICHARD C. SENELICK, M.D. is the Medical Director at the Rehabilitation Institute of San Antonio (RIOSA). He also serves as Program Director of the Head Injury and Stroke programs. A native of Illinois, Dr. Senelick did his undergraduate and medical school training at the University of Illinois in Chicago. A neurologist who specializes in neurorehabilitation, he subsequently completed his neurology training at the University of Utah in Salt Lake City. He served as a staff neurologist in the Air Force at Wilford Hall Medical Center for two years. He has authored numerous publications and co-authored a text book on visual physiology.

Dr. Senelick is Board Certified in neurology and a member of the American Academy of Neurology Section of Neurorehabilitation, American Congress of Rehabilitation Medicine, National Head Injury Foundation and the American Academy of Medical Directors.

CATHY E. RYAN, M.A., CCC-SLP, has served as the Program Director of the Head Injury and Stroke Programs at the Rehabilitation Institute of San Antonio. Ms. Ryan is a certified and licensed speech-language pathologist with over eight years experience in head injury rehabilitation. She has developed clinical programs for inpatient and outpatient head injury rehabilitation, as well as educational and support programs for family members and survivors.

Ms. Ryan received a masters degree in speech pathology from Northern Illinois University and earned a bachelor of science degree in Communicative Disorders from the University of Wisconsin-Madison.